"One problem that fertility specialists have is recommending a good book to help patients understand and manage their fertility. That problem has just been solved with *Dr. Robert Greene's Perfect Hormone Balance for Fertility.* This book is an 'on target' potpourri of details delivered in a readily accessible manner . . . it belongs in the hands of all couples experiencing the emotional and physical challenges of infertility."

—JOSEPH SANFILIPPO, M.D.,
past president, American Society
for Reproductive Medicine

"Dr. Robert Greene and Ms. Laurie Tarkan are to be congratulated for creating such a superb piece of work. *Perfect Hormone Balance for Fertility* provides the challenged consumer with loads of important evidence-based information, filling a huge void in this field of study. Every page of this book provides valuable and concise information that is stripped of confusing jargon for the average patient. I strongly endorse this book and will certainly recommend it to my patients as a 'must read'!"

of the
tive Medicine

"Dr. ontains a
pleth al sugges-
tion ving or is
alre

r for

Also by Dr. Robert Greene

Dr. Robert Greene's Perfect Balance
Dr. Robert Greene's Perfect Hormone Balance for Pregnancy
Happy Baby, Healthy Mom Pregnancy Journal

DR. ROBERT GREENE'S
PERFECT HORMONE BALANCE
FOR FERTILITY
The Ultimate Guide to Getting Pregnant

ROBERT A. GREENE, M.D., and LAURIE TARKAN

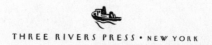

THREE RIVERS PRESS • NEW YORK

Copyright © 2008 by Robert A. Greene, M.D., and Laurie Tarkan

All rights reserved.
Published in the United States by Three Rivers Press, an imprint of the Crown Publishing Group, a division of Random House, Inc., New York.
www.crownpublishing.com

Three Rivers Press and the Tugboat design are registered trademarks of Random House, Inc.

Library of Congress Cataloging-in-Publication Data

Greene, Robert A.
    Dr. Robert Greene's perfect hormone balance for fertility : the ultimate guide to getting pregnant / Robert A. Greene and Laurie Tarkan.—1st ed.
    Includes bibliographical references and index.
1. Endocrine gynecology—Popular works.   2. Hormones—Popular works.
3. Fertility, Human—Popular works.   4. Women—Health and hygiene—Popular works.
I. Tarkan, Laurie.   II. Title.
    RG159.G73 2008
    618.1—dc22   2007027904

ISBN 978-0-307-33740-5

Printed in the United States of America

Design by Dominika Dmytrowski

Illustrations by Gail Tarkan Shube

10 9 8 7 6 5 4 3 2

First Edition

For Aevry

CONTENTS

DR. ROBERT GREENE'S
PERFECT HORMONE BALANCE
FOR FERTILITY

INTRODUCTION

When I started writing this book, my wife, Morgan, and I were going through fertility treatment ourselves. When we finally did get pregnant—and stayed pregnant—it was at a time in our lives that we were both following the Perfect Balance Fertility Program to a tee. Our personal experience—and our beautiful baby girl—reaffirmed for me the importance of my whole body approach to fertility and the evidence-based recommendations I offer in this book. First, let me share with you our story.

For years, we were very happy and content with our life together. In fact, with Einstein, DaVinci, KatMandu, and Lola—our two dogs and two cats—our house felt quite full of life. We had become immune to the question "When are you going to have kids?" which came at us from all angles—friends, family members, my patients, and my staff. In retrospect, I think what stiffened our resolve not to have children was fear—Morgan had an inner sense that she might have trouble getting pregnant, so it was easier for us to not confront the issue. After some time, though, we began to reconsider our vision of our family and face our fears, and decided that we truly wanted to have children together. We proceeded cautiously, with one foot in and one foot out, perhaps as a way of not letting our hopes get too high, or setting ourselves up for disappointment.

We chose not to tell anyone we were trying to have children for two reasons: it made it easier for us to walk away if things weren't going well, and we didn't want to raise the hopes of our family and then disappoint them. Last, to be honest, as a reproductive endocrinologist, I was a bit worried about how it would affect my patients if we could not get pregnant ourselves.

Given my medical specialty, we had a good idea of what our obstacles would be. The first potential problem was Morgan's age. She was 39 but was healthy, fit, active, and had no health complaints. For years, Morgan and I have lived the Perfect Balance diet plan that I recommend in this book. I, at 41, was also in good shape and practiced yoga. But just to be sure that our outward appearances reflected our inner health, Morgan had a blood test that confirmed that her ovaries were healthy, and I had a semen analysis that found no obvious problems.

The second potential obstacle, though more of a practical matter, seemed more insurmountable. I give lectures around the country on a weekly basis, easily placing me out of town several days each week, often when Morgan was ovulating. After several months of dealing with this frustration, we decided to use ovulation-enhancement medication in order to time Morgan's ovulation dates to when we would be together. I have used this approach with numerous patients who had similar work-life conflicts (in any case, I often recommend ovulation enhancement for women over 38).

Morgan began taking the drug Clomid to stimulate her ovaries, and on the very first treatment cycle, she got pregnant. We were very surprised because of our initial doubts. It almost seemed too easy. And it was—seven weeks into her pregnancy, Morgan miscarried. We were devastated. Morgan was just beginning to embrace her pregnancy, along with its symptoms, and the reality that she was indeed able to carry a child. But when the symptoms stopped and she miscarried, it seemed to confirm her own fears about her fertility. Since we never told anyone we were trying to get pregnant, we couldn't tell anyone when the pregnancy failed, which left us feeling very isolated.

Over the following nine months, we completed three cycles of ovulation enhancement. We had moved up the fertility treatment ladder, switching to an injectable medication that tends to be more successful than Clomid. We also started intrauterine insemination, in which I provided a specimen and my sperm were placed directly into Morgan's uterus when she was ovulating. We struck out.

As the eternal optimist, I knew we would become pregnant and wanted to push forward to the next level, which was in vitro fertilization (IVF). Morgan, of course, bore the brunt of the treatment—having to get hormone injections, the regular monitoring of her hormones, and then going through two surgical procedures: one to retrieve her eggs, and one to have two embryos placed back into her uterus.

She did not get pregnant. At that point, we felt we needed a break. Morgan found the monthly "cycle watch" emotionally exhausting. When we first started out, Morgan said she was not going to let this become an obsession for her, as she'd seen it happen with so many of our patients (she is a registered nurse who has worked with infertility patients). But it had started to become all-consuming. The fertility center wanted us to up our treatment to the next rung on the ladder, but she wanted to step back down and bring some balance back into her life. She tried to reduce her stress and started doing yoga.

When we were ready to start up again, we went back to basic ovulation enhancement—nothing high tech—and Morgan became pregnant at the age of 41. In the end, I believe it was the balance we sought after the failed IVF cycle that helped her to become pregnant, have a healthy pregnancy, and give birth to our baby girl. This balance is what I try to help all of my patients achieve.

◆   ◆   ◆

"What's wrong with us?" is the first question on the minds of most of my patients who are having trouble becoming pregnant. The thought that our bodies are somehow failing us in this essential human experience can make us feel helpless and out of control, and leave us grasping for reasons. Some couples begin to question the choices they've made in their lives, like delaying having a family or having used contraception earlier in their lives, and many start searching for answers—a diagnosis, something that can be fixed, a hormone that can be tweaked.

Though these thoughts and feelings are absolutely normal, I think there's a more hopeful way of approaching your fertility. I have seen in patient after patient, and in study after study, that fertility issues are not usually caused by one particular event or problem—even when there is a definitive diagnosis—but instead by many aspects of your health and well-being, those of your partner, and issues that arise when your body and your partner's interact with each other. This is the main reason why many couples who do attempt to be diagnosed are told they have "unexplained infertility." In the search to find that elusive diagnosis or best treatment, what often gets overlooked is basic *hormone balance.* And yet, nothing has a greater impact on your fertility, the success of your pregnancy, and the health of your child.

You have more than 100 hormones circulating in your body—reproductive hormones, pregnancy hormones, sex hormones, metabolic hormones, and stress hormones—relaying messages from tissue to tissue, organ to organ, brain to body, and body to brain. Their equilibrium— their *perfect balance*—determines your ability to conceive and support a pregnancy. The most current research clearly shows that when your body is not balanced, your brain may shut down one of the many links in the hormonal chain of events that leads to conception and having a healthy baby.

Imbalances can be corrected. That is very encouraging news.

As a fertility specialist, a reproductive endocrinologist, an obstetrician and gynecologist, as well as a hormone researcher, I have developed a philosophy along with an evidence-based lifestyle program that every couple or single person embarking on parenthood can follow to enhance their fertility. It is a program you can turn to if you and your partner are trying to become pregnant on your own, if you've been consulting with your obstetrician, or if you have already begun treatments with a fertility specialist. It is also essential reading for all couples that want to become pregnant, even if you haven't encountered any fertility frustrations, because hormone balance plays a critical role in preventing complications during pregnancy.

Perfect Hormone Balance for Fertility is based on the latest research from the fields of reproductive endocrinology and *neuroendocrinology,* the study of how hormones interact with your brain—what I call the *hormone-brain connection.* The research has painted a clear picture of how this hormone-brain connection impacts your fertility and how hormonal imbalances can create obstacles to fertility. Your brain, and more specifically, your *hypothalamus* (located in the central core of your brain), is your hormone control center, monitoring the interactions of hormones and their effects on your physiology. The hypothalamus also makes adjustments when it senses an imbalance, and these shifts can provoke symptoms and even create obstacles to becoming pregnant. The fact that imbalances often go undiagnosed and untreated is one important reason why success rates at fertility centers have reached a plateau in the past five to six years. Hormonal imbalance remains an untreated hurdle to higher success rates. Correcting imbalances could push the success rates even higher. Indeed, more and more countries are moving away from fertility treatments that rely on implanting multiple embryos into a woman's uterus to overcome fertility, as this approach often results in risky multiple pregnancies. They are beginning to explore the reality that lifestyle factors that affect your hormone balance play a major role in your ability to get pregnant. Their attention has shifted to ways to improve fertility without treatment and alongside of treatment. In this country, we are a few steps behind.

As a specialist who often sees patients who have not had success with other fertility doctors, I am surprised at how few of these couples have been told to improve their hormone balance as a way of improving their fertility. In the highly competitive world of fertility care, there is a strong tendency to attract couples ready for treatment and to jump directly into expensive treatments. Many well-intending health care providers fear losing the attention of their patients by telling them to take three to six months to address their lifestyle before entering active treatment. Yet, this is the amount of time it can take for many people to bring their hormones into a state of balance to raise their chance of conceiving.

Some of my patients who have come to me after being unsuccessfully treated with sophisticated assisted reproductive technologies (ARTs) such as IVF are often skeptical when I start asking them about how they feel, and probe them about seemingly unrelated symptoms. Are you tired? Have you been gaining weight? Is your partner depressed or stressed out? Has your libido weakened? Do you experience anxiety? We seem to have more faith in medical procedures than our own bodies. But symptoms matter! They speak volumes about your body's health and your hormone balance.

I personally understand how difficult it can be to step away from fertility procedures and look at how your own lifestyle is affecting your fertility. This is the choice Morgan and I made, and it took patience on

Case in Point

Laura and her husband Marcus, both in their late 20s, had been trying to conceive for two years. During that time, they underwent five cycles of fertility treatment, including IVF, without success. Laura had become depressed and they both were disappointed and cynical from their prior experiences. They were also doubtful when I began asking questions about Laura's diet and lifestyle, how she was feeling, and how optimistic she was that they'd succeed in having a baby.

She reported that she was gaining weight despite her frequent workouts, she felt tired and hopeless, and her periods were infrequent. I suspected that she had polycystic ovarian syndrome, or PCOS, a common hormonal problem that often goes undiagnosed—as it did for Laura. The hallmark of PCOS is insulin resistance, when cells become desensitized to the effects of insulin, a metabolic hormone that normally moves blood sugar out of the bloodstream and into cells for use as energy or fat storage. Insulin resistance leads to high insulin levels, which can affect the quality of eggs. She also had high levels of the stress hormone, cortisol, which is associated with depression.

We put Laura on the Perfect Balance program and recommended she make healthier food choices to lower her insulin resistance. She also made changes to her lifestyle to reduce her stress. Although she began feeling better and losing weight, I needed to put her on metformin (a medication typically used to treat diabetes because it makes your body respond more effectively to insulin). It is a pregnancy category B drug, which means that thousands of women have taken this during pregnancy without any increase in birth defects. Within a few weeks, it became even easier for Laura to lose weight. She told me her depression had lifted and she was starting to feel healthy. During the next four months, her menstrual cycles became regular, and by the 11th month, she had lost 20 pounds and was pregnant. No fertility treatment was necessary.

our parts. We opted to not do another IVF treatment, but to go back to simple ovulation induction, while, at the same time, Morgan tried to reduce the stress in her life through yoga. I have seen many patients who have had several unsuccessful attempts with IVF get pregnant after they stepped off the fertility treadmill and began to focus on balancing their hormones first.

Along with couples who may need to take a step back from fertility treatments, there are many couples who have decided not to pursue fertility treatments and those that have abandoned the idea of having a biological child. Only about one-third of couples experiencing fertility problems ever seek treatment. If you fall into these groups, you may become pregnant simply by balancing your hormones.

You probably have some intuitive understanding of the importance of hormonal balance on your fertility. Most of my patients, unprompted, tell me about their levels of stress or their attempts at relaxation in order to help them conceive. They suspect that high levels of stress hormones may negatively impact their fertility. The brain imaging research firmly supports their intuition. Stress hormones send messages to the brain that can prevent the release of pregnancy hormones, which in turn can prevent conception or raise the risk of miscarriage.

But stress hormones are just the tip of the iceberg. Of your many hormones, about a dozen or so directly affect your reproduction, and these are the ones that you are most likely to hear about if you go for fertility assessment and treatment. These hormones are indeed critical to your fertility, but they do not act alone. Hormones such as insulin, thyroid hormones, and sex hormones, as well as hormone-disrupting chemicals in the environment, can impair a woman's ability to release an egg, conceive, or stay pregnant. There are also hormones that affect a man's ability to produce abundant, high-quality sperm, or even maintain his sexual functioning. Male problems are responsible for at least one-third of infertility experienced by couples.

That's why simply injecting the egg-promoting hormone called follicle-stimulating hormone (FSH) as a fertility treatment—a typical approach—isn't necessarily going to make you pregnant. When I treat a couple, not only do I want to improve FSH levels, I want to make sure insulin levels are down, I want to get stress hormones back to normal, I want to make sure thyroid levels are just right, and I want to avoid high levels of the female hormone estrogen, and low levels of progesterone, a hormone that is essential in helping the uterus support a pregnancy.

Over the last 50 years, the rate of couples experiencing infertility has steadily risen to about one in five today. In only 7 years, between 1995 and 2002, the numbers increased by 20 percent from 6.1 million to 7.3 million. This frightening trend is partly attributed to our less-than-healthy lifestyles—having poor nutrition, eating fast foods, being overweight, being stressed out, not having enough time for sleep, leading inactive lives, and being exposed to hormone-disrupting chemicals and pollutants in our environment and our homes. Each of these factors has been shown to create hormonal imbalances that impact fertility. For example, studies show that having a diet high in simple carbohydrates lowers fertility by raising insulin levels, poor sleep can interfere with your brain's signal to promote your egg's release, and high stress hormone levels can block a fertilized egg from implanting correctly in your womb. Common pollutants, what I call *BioMutagens,* such as weed killer can lower your partner's sperm count, and second-hand cigarette smoke can lower your estrogen level, reducing the responsiveness of your ovaries and harming the quality of your eggs. Your whole body has to be in relative balance in order for these pregnancy hormones to function at their best. You can imagine, though, that even the most conscientious fertility specialist doesn't have time to address all these influences on your ability to conceive.

In this book, I will help you and your partner achieve healthy hormone balance and dramatically improve your chances of becoming pregnant.

TAKING CHARGE OF YOUR FERTILITY

Many of my patients tell me they feel helpless in the face of their fertility issues. If you have already experienced difficulty getting pregnant, you may feel confused about which direction you should turn—should you keep trying on your own, see your obstetrician, see a fertility specialist, start taking hormones, try acupuncture? Maybe you have already put your body through hormone treatments and assisted reproductive technologies at the recommendation of your doctors, but still haven't gotten pregnant. Or maybe you have given up on getting pregnant, assuming that high-tech fertility treatments are your only option—a path you don't want to go down. In any of these scenarios, you probably feel like you have little control over your body and your life plans.

Taking charge of your fertility is by far the best defense against feeling powerless and the most compelling reason for reading *Perfect Hormone Balance for Fertility.*

In this book, I will help you correct any imbalances you may have through my diet, exercise, and stress-busting recommendations. I will help you fully understand the factors that affect your fertility and how they influence your choices for treatment, if you choose to get treated.

Many obstetricians and fertility centers have a certain predetermined course of action, a *protocol* that they follow with all their patients. If A, then B; if not A, then C. But I believe that your fertility is as individual as your own DNA. This book will give you an individualized program to follow, and provide you with the knowledge to take an active role in your own treatment.

THE FERTILITY TRAPS

When a new couple comes to my practice and tells me their story, I often wish that I could have seen them years earlier. I feel frustrated that so many patients have undergone unnecessary tests and procedures, have repeated the same unsuccessful treatment month after month, or, on the other hand, were not given any valuable advice or treatments whatsoever, wasting their precious fertile years. Most have run into these typical problems with the way fertility issues are treated today.

First, too many women are rushed into assisted reproductive technologies, often when it's not necessary. I have seen how easily fertility doctors can get blinded by our technology and not think outside of the box. There can be almost an assembly line mentality. Some of the top fertility centers determine which treatment paradigms are most efficient and then develop protocols that they apply to groups of patients. Yet overall, less than 15 percent of all couples having fertility problems need IVF to successfully have their own biological children, but many more are encouraged to pursue this high-tech avenue. Not only is it unnecessary, but it's often unsuccessful because the underlying hormonal imbalances have not been addressed. I recommend taking a more individualized approach to diagnosing, correcting, and, when necessary, treating fertility problems—one that requires your active participation in the decision making.

But one of the most vexing and unfortunately common problems with doctors who treat fertility patients is their focus on how to produce more eggs and more embryos. In effect, they try to compensate for a hormonal deficiency by creating a hormonal overdose—one that produces too many eggs. The consequence has been a steady rise in the number of twins, triplets, and even greater multiple pregnancies. These pregnancies often put women into even more hormone chaos because each individually developing fetus creates higher levels of hormones than that of a single pregnancy. This leads to a higher rate of preterm labor, cesarean section, and pregnancy complications like preeclampsia—all a result of not achieving balance. It also puts the developing fetuses at risk. Too often women carrying three or more embryos, the earliest stage of development, also face the devastating choice of whether they should have a "reduction," a procedure that compromises one or more embryos so the others have a better chance of survival and good health. I have helped many couples avoid multiple pregnancies by first bringing a person into hormonal balance so that fewer eggs are needed for success.

One major difference between most fertility doctors and myself is that they focus on working around your problem, whereas I seek to correct the underlying hormonal problems or at least optimize hormonal balance first. For example, if I can identify why a woman isn't ovulating and correct the underlying problem, then I don't have to prescribe medications that force her to produce and release multiple eggs. I make sure that I diagnose before I treat (many fertility centers rush straight to treatment), and I rarely recommend a fertility treatment without having a firm grasp on what hormonal imbalance is in play. I focus my practice on doing everything I can to help women become pregnant *without* using IVF or other ARTs. When necessary, I absolutely recommend an ART, but many of my patients get pregnant without it.

ACHIEVING PERFECT BALANCE

In Part One, I will provide you with a solid understanding of the hormonal issues that can affect your fertility. I'll discuss how your and your partner's reproductive systems function, and how your lifestyles affect their peak functioning.

In Part Two, the Perfect Balance Fertility Program, I will help bring your body into hormonal balance through recommendations for nutrition, exercise, stress reduction, BioMutagen avoidance, and other lifestyle changes. I will also recommend checkups and tests you should complete now to make sure you don't have any underlying health problems that might interfere with your fertility or pregnancy. And I will provide you with the first steps you can take at home to improve your success rates, as well as help you pull together the information you need for your first consultation if you choose to go this route.

In Part Three, I will review all the issues that may affect your chance of success—your so-called *fertility factors,* which are typically reviewed as part of a normal fertility evaluation. But I go one step further than most evaluations and provide you with a system to rate your fertility factors, so you can understand how mild or serious each factor is, allowing you to make smarter decisions about your treatment. I will also provide detailed questionnaires and specific recommendations for tests so that you and your doctor can better diagnose your fertility factors, and to help you avoid delays or costly detours to success. I also provide questionnaires for your partner because I believe you both need to be fully engaged in the evaluation, decision making, and treatment.

In Part Four, I guide you through all the treatment options and make recommendations for which treatments may be most appropriate for you, based on your fertility factors and personal preferences. I will advise you about how to navigate the latest advanced fertility techniques and the "alphabet soup" of acronyms used to describe them. I will also recommend acupuncture, yoga, and other complementary practices that are proven to increase your chance of success. I will also offer options on prolonging your fertility through high-tech measures. Depending on your age, current medical conditions, or your social situation, you might want to explore freezing eggs, sperm, or embryos to give you healthy options for the future.

A threat to your fertility brings up so many intense emotions, and these emotions can have a profound impact on your ability to make decisions. Couples with fertility issues may be among the most vulnerable patients, willing to try anything and spend any amount of money to be able to carry a baby to term. My goal in writing this book is to help you explore what changes you can make to improve your own fertility as well as to provide the information you need to make the best choices for yourself and future family. My recommendations are based on the latest scientific research that appears in the top peer-reviewed medical journals. I include study references that back up these recommendations and I encourage you to bring this book—along with the reference list—to your health care provider, so that you establish a healthy partnership in your quest for a baby.

1

Fertility and Your Hormones

1 Hormone Balance: The Foundation of Fertility

I have no doubt that the rising incidence of hormone imbalance is behind the steady rise in infertility. Our diet, lifestyle, and work habits have all changed in ways that invite or even create these imbalances. Because of our busy schedules, we gravitate toward fast foods and prepackaged meals that are high in unhealthy carbohydrates and fats. Eating poorly can easily lead to hormonal chaos, reducing your chance of conception or increasing your risk of pregnancy complications. We've also become less active, and some of us, completely sedentary, and we accept stress and a lack of sleep as a part of life. Yet better food choices, regular exercise, adequate rest, and stress-reducing activities can improve your health enormously and enhance your ability to conceive.

We are also exposed to a growing number of chemicals each year through our food, air, water, cleaning products, gardening chemicals, and personal care products. Some people are also exposed to more chemicals at work. Fertility and hormone specialists have become increasingly concerned about these chemicals because many have the ability to disrupt your own hormone functions, which in

Did you know ?

Perfect Balance describes that sensation when you feel great, function at your peak levels, and even look your best.

Fertility Fact

Birth Spacing and Secondary Infertility

Timing may be important for couples experiencing secondary infertility. "Birth spacing" refers to planning the ideal interval between pregnancies. Along with thinking about how far apart you want your kids to be in age, you need to think about hormonal balance. It takes time after childbirth for your nutritional status to improve enough to support another pregnancy. It takes time for your body to reestablish hormonal balance. But if you wait *too* long, your reproductive hormones may fall out of balance. A recent analysis of 67 studies looking at the outcomes of more than 11 million pregnancies demonstrated that the ideal interval between pregnancies is between 18 months and 6 years. Waiting fewer than 18 months resulted in a much higher risk of preterm birth or having a baby with low birth weight. Women who waited only 6 months also had a higher risk of miscarriage. Couples, especially those who remarry, might want to keep the 6-year mark in mind when planning to expand their family together.

turn can affect your fertility. These chemicals also may contribute to miscarriage or compromise the health of your baby. But in many cases you can restore hormone harmony through simple changes in your lifestyle, and, in so doing, you will improve your fertility, your health, and your well-being.

THE HORMONE DANCE

Your hormones are constantly shifting based on what is happening in your body on any given day. Each organ and each system has its own agenda, sending out hormonal signals to alert the others and elicit their cooperation. For instance, your digestive system calls upon your circulatory system for more blood flow after a meal to help distribute fuel and nutrients throughout your body. On the other hand, if you're under stress, hormones will shift your blood flow away from your digestive system and direct it to your muscles to prepare you for dealing with the danger at hand. Your brain's hypothalamus is at the helm, listening in on all the hormone cross talk and prioritizing messages, so that you're not falling asleep when you sit down to eat, perspiring when your body temperature is low, or menstruating when a fertilized egg is trying to implant in your womb.

Your brain also initiates many bodily events, often in response to what you're experiencing or what's going on hormonally. If you're frightened, your brain sends hormonal messages that override other biological functions like sleepiness or hunger. When you're sexually aroused, your brain sends hormones that signal your body to prepare for intimate acts. If you're determined to complete a task, your brain sends pick-me-up hormones to fend off fatigue. And if your body doesn't have enough stored calories to support a pregnancy, your brain blocks signals to your ovaries—effectively preventing ovulation. The hormone-brain connection is the key to understanding why achieving hormonal balance is necessary to improve your chances of conception and having a healthy baby.

It is equally important for couples who have had a baby but are having difficulty conceiving again, a condition called *secondary infertility*. Many of these couples have developed a hormone imbalance since the delivery of their last child. The imbalance is what is keeping them from becoming pregnant again. Before jumping into treatment, these couples need to consider the importance of their hormones and how their diet, weight, lifestyle, or health may have changed in the intervening years.

Because there are so many hormones, and many that have similar jobs, I like to group them together based on their functions. Each of the four groups I have identified needs to be in a state of equilibrium. I like to think of these groups as the elements of a mobile, with the brain at the pinnacle monitoring your dynamic state of hormone balance.

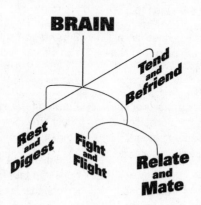

When subtle imbalances occur within a group, they might not disrupt the other groups. For example, your hypothalamus might make minor adjustments to your levels of estrogen and progesterone, keeping them in relative balance and not adversely affecting your fertility. But if one hormone gets too high or too low, and the others can't balance it out, then this discordance can affect the other hormone groups and disrupt your health completely—especially your fertility. Since conception and reproduction are not essential for your survival, I place these hormones in the most vulnerable position of the mobile to reflect their reliance on everything else being near perfect. Below are the four categories of hormones and what they do, how they interact, and how they affect your fertility. Please note that I will provide descriptions and details on all of these hormones later in the book.

1. **Rest-and-digest hormones** (key hormones include insulin, leptin, growth hormone, ghrelin, and melatonin). This group controls growth, digestion, and weight, as well as repair and rejuvenation. Because of their role in weight gain and loss, imbalances can lead to obesity, diabetes, and a host of related diseases. I will focus a great deal on this group in the program since your weight and the

PERFECT BALANCE HORMONE BIOSYSTEM

Many hormones are available in supplements and medications. I've devised a system to help you understand how they work and how they differ from one another. You'll encounter these terms throughout the book, and I will explain them in more detail in the treatment section, where I describe hormone therapies that are used in treatment.

◆ **BioIdentical** hormones are so close to your body's naturally produced hormones that your brain can't tell the difference.

◆ **BioSimilar** hormones are similar but not identical to your hormones and may offer some advantages over BioIdentical hormones in certain circumstances.

◆ **BioLimited** hormones are designed to replicate some functions of your own hormones, while limiting the functions of others.

◆ **BioAntagonist** hormones effectively turn off your natural hormones and are used to control or prevent disease like breast cancer.

◆ **BioModifiers** are medications that affect the way your body responds to hormones.

◆ **BioUnknowns** are hormone preparations (typically found in herbal supplements) that act in ways that are still unknown.

◆ **BioMutagens** are not therapies, but are toxic chemicals in the environment that disrupt your hormones.

balance of these hormones have an enormous impact on your fertility, and because you have some control over them. There are clear and effective steps you can take to restore their balance, including making better food choices.

2. **Tend-and-befriend hormones** (key hormones include thyroid hormone, prolactin, and diuretic hormones like aldosterone). This group is in charge of tending to your body's basic physiological needs, such as maintaining your temperature and hydration, and meeting your oxygen needs. Some of these hormones, like prolactin, also impact your emotional bonding with others. Imbalances, though, can make you more susceptible to infections, less able to turn off your stress response, less adaptable to temperature and altitude changes, and can put you at a higher risk of disorders like chronic fatigue and anemia. When tend-and-befriend hormones are out of sync, they shift your body's resources away from reproduction, contributing to infertility.

3. **Fight-and-flight hormones** (key hormones are adrenaline, cortisol, endorphins, and corticotropin releasing hormone). These are the well-known stress hormones, released when you believe you're in danger or your health is threatened. They help redirect necessary resources toward survival against an imminent threat or a perceived hazard that may not even exist. When stress hormones are chronically elevated, you may experience depression, anxiety, sleep disorders, or chronic pain, and you may have difficulty getting pregnant. To your stressed body, pregnancy is one more major challenge, or stressor, so to "protect" you, your brain halts all events and hormonal triggers geared toward conceiving.

4. **Relate-and-mate hormones** (key hormones are estrogen, testosterone, progesterone, follicle-stimulating hormone (FSH), and luteinizing hormone (LH). These sex and pregnancy hormones are the most important hormones for fertility and reproduction. They guide the production and release of fertile eggs and healthy sperm. They also play a role in cementing the bonds of your intimate relationships with your sexual partner as well as with your children— these are more potent bonding agents than the tend-and-befriend hormones. Imbalances in this group are the most obvious ones to

consider when diagnosing infertility. They can interfere with the growth and release of a mature egg each month or cause a low sperm count in your partner, or even affect how successfully the fertilized egg implants in your uterus. Imbalances can also cause sexual dysfunction, such as low libido and erectile dysfunction or pain associated with sex.

Partner Pointer

Your Hormone-Brain Connection Matters, Too

Though you may not have realized it, your relationship and even your goal of becoming a father creates hormonal shifts in you that affect how you feel and how you interact with others. Your hormone-brain connection is far subtler than the changes that women go through, but it's nonetheless real—and measurable. For instance, levels of testosterone, the hormone that drives libido and competitiveness, are highest in the morning. It's no coincidence that most women ovulate in the middle of the night and will have their eggs in perfect position for fertilization by the time you wake up. Interestingly, men in stable relationships and fathers wake up with testosterone levels that are identical to those of single men, yet by early evening, their levels of testosterone lag behind those without partners—a physiological response that may keep the attached male closer to home in the evening. So consider planning for some intimate moments in the morning before work rather than at the end of the day, when your libido has waned.

SYMPTOMS MATTER!

Many doctors often forget to ask their fertility patients the basic question: "How are you feeling?" Or if they ask, they don't listen carefully to the answer. Yet, that's the information that I find most revealing because it's the best indicator of whether your hormones are in a state of equilibrium. This idea of considering your symptoms when looking at fertility issues is just now beginning to catch on in the medical community. It is well supported by brain imaging research showing how hormone imbalances detected by your brain trigger symptoms throughout your body. We can correlate brain activity in precise areas of the brain to specific symptoms. For instance, chronic fatigue is associated with reduced hormone activity in the base of your brain, whereas anxiety is associated with an increase in activity in the area behind your forehead.

Case in Point

I first met Ally following a seminar I gave to a support group for obese patients considering gastric bypass surgery (this surgery creates a detour past some regions of the intestines in order to promote weight loss). At 34, Ally had given up on the idea of becoming pregnant. She and her husband had seen several fertility specialists and endured several failed treatments. She was repeatedly told to diet, and told her weight problem was simply due to her own behavior and lack of willpower. This added guilt to her worsening situation and had pushed her toward the gastric bypass surgery.

I knew immediately that her problems were caused by hormone imbalances. I told her that surgery must be combined with the Perfect Balance diet and lifestyle program to promote hormone balance. After several months following the program, Ally lost 30 pounds and her menstrual cycles became regular for the first time in her life. I recommended that she take a birth control pill, Yaz, until her hormones became more balanced. It's recommended that women wait at least 12 months after gastric bypass surgery before becoming pregnant. The birth control pill also placed her ovaries in a rested state as she continued to lose weight. After 6 months, she lost almost 80 pounds and felt she wanted to try to get pregnant. She was surprised when I recommended that rather than beginning fertility treatment, she simply stop her birth control pills and use a monitor to predict ovulation so she could time intercourse to her most fertile days. Ally conceived after only 4 more months, and delivered a healthy baby girl.

Symptoms will arise when your brain unsuccessfully attempts to correct hormone imbalances. Hormone-related symptoms are not always as obvious or easy to interpret as symptoms of the flu or an injury. They can be subtle, like an inability to stay asleep, or slow but steady unexplained weight gain. Yes, there are symptoms that appear to have a clear connection to fertility, such as abnormal menstrual cycles or recurrent miscarriages. But the symptoms that don't appear remotely related to your fertility may be the ones preventing you from becoming pregnant. Recall the hormone mobile and how imbalances in any one group can affect your fertility.

Being overweight is one of the most common symptoms of hormone imbalance, and it's a common cause of infertility. Overweight women who lose as little as 5 percent of their body weight can dramatically improve their fertility. When overweight men lose this much weight, it can boost their sperm count as well as their libido. But other symptoms are telling as well. If you suffer from insomnia, acne, depression, or even sexual dysfunction, these may be clues to hormone imbalances.

Focusing on how you and your partner have been feeling can help you gauge how close the both of you are to hormonal balance. Imbalances are by far the most common obstacles to pregnancy and among the most common reasons for miscarriage. Creating hormonal balance through changes in your diet, activity level, stress-reducing activities, and exposure to BioMutagens—all topics I discuss in Part Two—is the first step to improving your fertility, if not restoring it altogether.

Ask Dr. Greene

Q Do age-related hormone changes affect my chances of having twins?

A Yes, if your hormonal balance is tipped in favor of egg promotion, it can increase your chance of twins. Women who become pregnant in their late 30s or early 40s are almost twice as likely to have twins as women in their early 20s (this increase is independent of the use of fertility treatments, which increases the chances even more). FSH, which prepares your eggs for ovulation, rises as you age, and is the cause for this higher twin rate.

2 Protecting Your Fertility

Balancing your hormones to improve your reproductive health is a whole-body approach that has an impact on all levels of your reproductive process. It affects the genetic code (DNA) of your eggs and your partner's sperm, the hormones that stimulate their development, whether egg and sperm meet up, and if the fertilized egg, or embryo, can implant in your uterus. So before you progress to the nuts and bolts of my program, I want to provide you with a general understanding of the reproductive process—specifically, the journey your eggs and your partner's sperm take through your lifetimes. If you are in the midst of or on the threshold of fertility treatment, refer to chapters 8 and 9 for more detailed accounts of the life cycle of sperm and eggs.

GAZILLIONS OF SPERM

With every heartbeat, a man produces about 1,500 microscopic sperm, and with each ejaculation, he typically releases over 20 million. This prolific production continues for 50 to 60 years, but it is fraught with imperfections. Every sperm develops out of a primitive cell, called a *spermatagonium,* which, like all other cells in the human body, has 46 chromosomes—23 pairs containing the DNA, or genetic code, that is necessary for the body to function. To become a mature sperm that can fertilize an egg, a spermatagonium has to shed one chromosome from each pair (your egg goes through the same process just before ovulation), so that when egg and sperm come together, their DNA will form 23 new pairs of chromosomes that will create a unique being—your child. In men, the process of maturation is called *spermatogenesis,* and takes about 90 days to complete.

During this time, sperm are highly susceptible to damage. They divide so rapidly, generating heat with each division, that they require the outer-body home of the testicles to keep cool. High temperatures—from a hot tub or a sauna—can make them more susceptible to genetic damage and slight imperfections. They are also highly vulnerable to hormonal imbalances and nutritional deficiencies. Sperm analysis studies have shown that in fertile men as few as 12 percent of sperm meet certain strict criteria—based upon their size, shape, and appearance—to be considered normal. Many sperm will have structural problems or minor flaws in their DNA, some of which are caused by hormonal imbalances and exposure to pollutants. Sperm are also unable to store energy and have a very limited life span. Many of the recommendations in my Perfect Balance program are aimed at creating hormone balance in order to minimize DNA damage to sperm and developing eggs.

Ask Dr. Greene

Q Do men have a "biological clock"?

A As men age, subtle changes in their sperm's DNA increase the risk of miscarriage as well as problems like autism in their offspring. With age, men also lose *Leydig* cells, helper cells that support developing sperm by providing calories, making hormones, and eliminating waste. As Leydig cells are lost, the testicles become less effective at making sperm, resulting in a gradual drop in sperm count and reduction in fertility beginning around age 40.

AN EGG'S RISE TO DOMINANCE—AND OVULATION

Compared to the billions of sperm your partner produces, you will ovulate about 400 eggs in your lifetime. A mature egg, called an *oocyte* (pronounced oh-oh-site) is one of the largest cells in a woman's body—about the size of the period at the end of this sentence (sperm are microscopic and some of the smallest cells in a man's body). While sperm are solitary cells that often travel in packs but abide by the credo "every sperm for himself," each oocyte is like a queen with its own attached entourage of handmaidens that provide hormones and nutrients to the maturing egg. Sounds like a cooperative system, but each month several queens compete for dominance over the others. Ovulation is a competitive process.

It takes about 290 days for each egg to come out of dormancy, complete maturation, and be readied for release. Like male sperm, an immature egg has to lose one copy of each of its 23 pairs of chromosome. Each month, the competitive race begins among a dozen or so activated eggs that simultaneously begin making genetic and metabolic changes to prepare themselves for ovulation. A few eggs begin to dominate and release hormones that halt the maturation of the other eggs in their group. Eventually, one egg (occasionally two) wins the contest and is prepared for ovulation, while the other eggs atrophy.

Did you know ?

When you were a 12-week-old fetus, the immature eggs contained in your teeny ovaries peaked at about 6 to 7 million. From that moment, they began their decline, so that by the time you were born, you had *only* 2 million left. When you had your first menstrual cycle, you were down to about 500,000—though that is more than enough to maintain your fertility well into your forties.

DIFFERENCES AND SIMILARITIES IN MALE AND FEMALE REPRODUCTION

	Women	Men
Number of chromosomes	46	46
Sex chromosomes	XX	XY
Number of immature eggs and sperm (gametes)	Fixed at birth. Numbers gradually fall throughout reproductive years.	Continuously produced from puberty through eighth decade of life.
Time for gametes to mature	About 290 days for an egg to mature and become fertile	90 days for sperm to mature and become fertile
Reproduction pattern	Monthly cycle	Continuous daily production
Window of conception	Egg remains fertile for about one day after release.	Sperm remain fertile for about five days after ejaculation.
Biological clock	Fertility declines noticeably at around age 35.	Fertility begins gradually declining around age 40.

The final two months in which these eggs are maturing and preparing for ovulation are an important time for your hormones to be in balance.

<table>
<tr><td>

Did you know **?**

As women reach their late 30s, more eggs are activated each month to begin the maturation process, meaning that more eggs die off each month, contributing to the reduced fertility experienced by women after age 35.

</td><td>

Your eggs are maturing rapidly and need a large supply of energy, nutrients, and hormones to help them function and mature properly. Hormonal imbalances during this time are a major contributor to infertility. Dramatic dieting or overexercising, for example, can limit the nutrients surrounding the egg and compromise egg development and maturation.

The longer an egg has waited in your ovaries, the more likely it is to encounter problems when it becomes activated, explaining the decrease in fertility experienced by women in their late reproductive

</td></tr>
</table>

years. By following the diet and lifestyle recommendations in my program, you can help protect and extend the health of your eggs.

FERTILIZATION AND IMPLANTATION

Having healthy eggs and viable sperm sets the stage for conception and a successful pregnancy, but it doesn't guarantee it. A couple considered *fertile* only has about a one in five chance of conception on any given month—assuming they have sex at the right time.

Immediately after your partner ejaculates during intercourse, his sperm forms a gel that covers your *cervix* (the canal that leads from your vagina to your uterus). The gel helps protect the sperm from being attacked by your immune system and from the normal acidity of the vagina. This acidity can damage vulnerable sperm, which are unable to repair themselves. So they have to get into your womb's more hospitable environment quickly in order to survive. On average, about 1 percent of sperm make it past the opening of the cervix—the rest die along the journey.

The next phase of the journey through the uterus to the *fallopian tubes* is fairly rapid—taking about 30 to 60 minutes. Yes, sperm are strong swimmers, but they also surf the wavelike contractions of your

Female Reproductive System

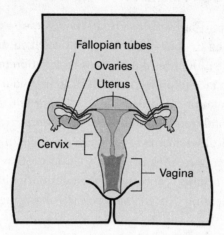

uterus that occur during orgasm. These contractions also point sperm in the direction of the ovary that released the egg. Any sperm remaining in the uterus after a few hours are probably attacked by immune cells, so it's crucial that they make it safely to the fallopian tubes.

Your tubes, two thin crayon-long canals, are like lush rain forests, protecting and nourishing the sperm, yet slowing their pace so they don't race to the end of the tube too quickly. Sperm can thrive in a tube for about five days after they arrive. Since the egg is only fertile for about one day after it is released, it's always better for sperm to arrive early and await the egg, rather than keep the egg waiting. Once ovulation occurs, the flared end of your fallopian tube acts almost like a catcher's mitt to enclose and receive the released egg. If all goes well, the egg will be fertilized by the sperm within the first centimeter of its journey toward your uterus.

As the DNA from your egg and your partner's sperm begins to meld together, the process of fertilization is complete and the fertilized egg, now called a *zygote,* is gently swept along by the beating motion of hairlike structures that line the tube. During this four to five day journey, its cells divide every few hours or so, until it arrives in your uterus, where it must implant into the *endometrium,* the uterine lining, which in turn provides it with nourishment and oxygen. Your pregnancy hormones support all of these phases of the journey and will guide the rest of the pregnancy.

PROTECTING YOUR FERTILITY

Your eggs and your partner's sperm are not immune to the chemicals that are circulating in your body. As I just described, their DNA is vulnerable to outside influences during their maturation process. But there are steps you can take to protect your DNA so that your eggs and sperm don't acquire mutations and degrade. It's important to avoid harmful chemicals and conditions throughout your reproductive years, but this is especially critical when you're trying to conceive. In addition to taking the preventive measures below, it's vital to follow the Perfect Balance program in order to consume all the necessary nutrients while the eggs you'll be releasing over the next year are maturing.

♀ For Her

No tobacco use. Up to 13 percent of all fertility problems are related to tobacco use. Women who smoke a pack of cigarettes a day tend to begin menopause several years earlier than nonsmokers. Tobacco is believed to accelerate the loss of eggs by damaging DNA and by its effect on estrogens. Tobacco smoke also makes it more difficult for an embryo to implant in the uterus following fertilization. In a study of IVF patients who received donated eggs, those who smoked had a 50 percent lower pregnancy rate and an increased risk of multiple births than nonsmokers. Recent evidence suggests that even second-hand smoke may carry a heavy risk as well. Before you attempt fertility treatments, talk to your doctor about trying one of the many safe and effective quitting methods now available.

Choose safe personal care products. Of the nearly 11,000 ingredients contained in cosmetics, only 11 percent have been evaluated for their safety by the cosmetics industry. The Food and Drug Administration (FDA) has not set safety standards for personal care products and does not require companies to test the safety of their products or inform consumers of the results when they do—even when found to be unsafe. It is essentially a self-regulated $50 billion industry. Consequently, unlimited amounts of potentially harmful chemicals are added to makeup, nail polish, perfumes, shampoos, hair sprays, deodorants, and so on. Some of the chemicals are known carcino-

ENDOMETRIOSIS AND ENVIRONMENTAL STRESS

An estimated 5 million women in the United States have endometriosis—a painful condition in which tissue from the endometrium travels to the ovary, fallopian tubes, and other surfaces in the pelvis. It also contributes to infertility (see chapter 12 for more information). Endometriosis researchers have been looking at links between environmental BioMutagens and this condition. The strongest associations have been found with dioxin and polychlorinated biphenyls (PCBs)—both toxic by-products of manufacturing and waste disposal plants. Studies show that women exposed to these chemicals have a three- to fourfold increased risk of developing endometriosis. Typically exposure occurs through contaminated air and water. This may be the strongest direct link between BioMutagens and a condition known to reduce fertility.

gens; others can cause birth defects or are potentially toxic to your reproductive health. You do not need to eschew these products altogether. Safer alternatives are available for use in cosmetics. See Appendix B, "BioMutagens in Cosmetics, Food, and the Environment" for a list of some of the most harmful products to avoid. You can also check out www.SafeCosmetics.org for more information.

Avoid other toxins. We are exposed to many BioMutagens on a regular basis through our food, water, air, and household and gardening products. Currently, there are about 80,000 chemicals used commercially in the United States with about 1,000 new ones added each year. Many of these chemicals wind up in the environment or in the products that we use despite the fact that only about 5 percent have ever been tested for their impact upon reproductive function. The Environmental Protection Agency (EPA) acknowledges that at least 50 of the commonly used chemicals they've tested affect reproduction in animals, but only four of them—lead, radiation, ethylene oxide, and dibromochloropropane—are regulated to monitor their safety and appropriate disposal. Many of these potentially hazardous chemicals are classified as endocrine or hormone disrupters. They can increase the rate of egg loss and reduce the ability of embryos to implant and develop. The list also includes weed killers, solvents, pesticides, and exhaust fumes. See Appendix B for a list of BioMutagens in your environment.

CONSIDER ORAL CONTRACEPTIVES WHEN NOT TRYING TO GET PREGNANT

Ongoing research suggests that use of hormone contraceptives may slow the rate of oocyte loss that occurs with aging, and may therefore delay menopause. According to the theory, birth control pills quiet the process of egg recruitment, so fewer eggs are activated and ultimately lost each cycle. The theory needs to be confirmed by further research. What we know for certain is that birth control pills don't compromise lifetime fertility and actually improve it during the months immediately after you go off of them. They can also lower your risk of cancer of the ovary, uterus, and colon, and do not raise the risk of breast cancer, as was once feared.

Avoid occupational BioMutagens. Many people are exposed to Bio-Mutagens in their workplace. As awareness continues to grow, certain occupations (auto mechanics, farmers, manicurists, firefighters, and dry-cleaning employees) have become more closely associated with low sperm count, recurrent miscarriage, or changes in menstrual cycles. Review Appendix B for a list of common agents associated with specific jobs. If you believe you're being exposed to any BioMutagens, your employer should be willing to reassign you to ensure your health and safety. Follow these general guidelines for avoiding occupational hazards, recommended by the Occupational Safety and Health Administration (OSHA):

◆ Dress accordingly to avoid skin contact with chemicals at work.
◆ Whenever appropriate, use protective gloves and goggles.
◆ Wash your hands thoroughly before eating or drinking at work.
◆ Wash potentially contaminated work clothes separately from household laundry and under recommended conditions.
◆ Participate in regular workplace safety training and education.
◆ Take precautionary steps to avoid airborne chemicals, bacteria, and viruses by working with properly designed airflow units—your employer should provide this information for you.

Use herbs and supplements with caution. Many herbs and supplements have ingredients that may compromise egg quality, disrupt ovulation, or cause miscarriage or premature birth. If they're poor-quality supplements, they may have contaminants that can harm a developing fetus. The FDA does not test supplements for effectiveness, and is just beginning to require manufacturers to ensure the products are pure and contain exactly what they claim on the label. Most supplements are not standardized, so each "dose" may not be the same. Talk to your doctor about the herbs and supplements you are taking or are considering during the critical months before you conceive.

Minimize pelvic surgeries or pelvic X-rays. Some doctors recommend surgery for ovarian cysts or pelvic pain, but surgery comes with the risk of scarring, reduced blood flow, and damage to healthy tissue. Avoid surgery by asking about alternatives like *expectant management*—the use of birth control pills or even temporary suppression of menstrual cycles to decrease the hormonal stimulation to the cysts, giving them time to heal.

♂ For Him

Avoid tobacco and marijuana. Using the legal and the illicit has been associated with reduced sperm count. Incidentally, smokeless tobacco may carry an even greater risk than cigarettes. If you need help quitting, talk to your doctor about the many safe and effective methods now available. If your partner smokes, try quitting together. Hormone-brain studies show it tends to be harder for women to quit, but the support could benefit both of you.

Keep it cool. Your testicles are located outside of your body because sperm need cooler temperatures (about 2 degrees or so less than your normal body temperature) to survive. Avoid hot tubs, saunas, tight clothing, laptops, or anything that can raise their temperature for extended periods of time.

Reevaluate your medications and supplements. Many different products have ingredients that may reduce sperm function or sperm count. For instance, calcium channel blockers, widely used to treat high blood pressure, can reduce a sperm's ability to penetrate an egg. Other drugs for gout, ulcers, or psoriasis are also known to reduce sperm function. There is even a Chinese herb called *thunder god vine,* or *lei gong ten,* that's been used to treat psoriasis, rheumatoid arthritis, liver disease, and fever, which has such a profound ability to inhibit sperm motility that it is being investigated as a form of male birth control. It's likely that other herbs that haven't been studied can also inhibit male fertility. Talk to your doctor about your medications and avoid supplements with ingredients that have not been well researched.

Avoid toxins at work and home. Many different toxins can compromise sperm count, such as weed killers, solvents, exhaust fumes, and X-rays. See Appendix B for a complete list and take extra steps to avoid unnecessary exposure.

Protect yourself against injury. Injuries can cause blood to leak out of your blood vessels, which can end up exposing your testicles to white blood cells. If they're exposed, you can develop an immune reaction to your own sperm. That's why trauma or even previous pelvic surgery can compromise male fertility. For instance, men who have had a vasectomy or hernia repair will often produce antibodies (small proteins) that attach to the tail of the sperm and impede their ability to swim.

Along with taking these precautions, you and your partner should undergo a number of preconception health exams to get a clean bill of health. These tests, which comprise your first step in the Perfect Balance Fertility Program, will help identify and reduce any potential obstacles to pregnancy.

2

Perfect Balance Fertility Program

Introduction: Balancing Your Hormones to Enhance Fertility

No matter where you are in your journey to fertility, you will benefit from hormone balance. The Perfect Balance Fertility Program is for all couples—from those of you who are just beginning to think about starting a family to those who have been through numerous treatment cycles, and everyone in between. The steps you take now will not only improve your fertility but will also improve how you feel once you're pregnant, improve the health of your developing baby, and reduce your complications during pregnancy.

This program is the result of over a decade and a half of my experience integrating the latest research in the care of couples challenged by fertility issues. I created this program to optimize your hormone balance, and your chance of success, even before you begin going through routine testing and diagnosis. By correcting your dietary hormone triggers, reducing your exposure to hormone-disrupting BioMutagens, and incorporating simple lifestyle adjustments, you may even conceive without any treatment at all. Many of my own patients who restored their hormone balance have gotten pregnant without any fertility treatments, and others responded to treatments that were previously unsuccessful for them.

The program begins with a chapter on preconception care, which focuses on getting your body prepared for pregnancy. I'll bring you and your partner up to date on all your general and reproductive health exams and everything else you should do before you start trying to become pregnant or start fertility treatments. If you've already initiated treatment, review my recommendations to make sure your preconception care has been complete. If you have existing medical conditions or are taking medications, I'll explain how you can minimize their effects on your fertility and pregnancy. In the chapters that follow, I'll provide a healthy nutritional plan that will help you maintain hormone balance, or correct any imbalances you may have, such as those associated with being overweight or underweight. I'll describe how a balanced fitness plan can improve your fertility—for underexercisers as well as hardcore athletes. I'll then provide one of the most important aspects of your fertility program—how to reduce the impact of stress hormone levels on your body. It's absolutely essential that you follow these recommendations to the best of your ability for at least three to six months in order to fully reap the hormone-balancing benefits. This pause in your journey might feel like an eternity, but it will significantly improve your chances of getting pregnant. You may begin to experience shifts in your hormone balance in only a couple of months, but don't be discouraged if it takes a little longer.

The program closes with a chapter on what you can do now to improve your chances of getting pregnant, such as monitoring your menstrual cycles and timing sex to the most fertile window of time in your cycle. I will also describe the first steps you should take if you decide you want to seek fertility treatment, if you want to change the course of your current treatment, or simply get a consultation. These include finding a specialist as well as drawing up a fertility plan. I'll help you pull together information on your medical history and family history to make that first visit productive and fruitful. With this information, you'll be several steps ahead of the game and will be able to have extremely informative discussions with your health care provider. You may be able to home in on what diagnostic tests you'll need, and more important, what diagnostic tests you don't want, saving you time, money, delays, and the aggravations of excessive and unnecessary testing.

3 Preconception Planning

If you are just embarking on expanding your family or are already trying to become pregnant, you now have the advantage of being able to plan for pregnancy. Leading experts agree that the mother's health *before* she becomes pregnant has a big impact on the health and well-being of her baby. Many medical associations from the American Academy of Pediatrics to the American College of Obstetricians and Gynecologists (ACOG) have written guidelines for preconception care, but according to a 2006 commission, only one in six health care providers offer preconception care to the majority of their patients. But one study found that nearly 85 percent of couples that have completed preconception planning would recommend it to others.

No matter where you are in your pursuit of pregnancy, you and your partner should follow these recommendations to improve your chances of conceiving and to minimize your risks of complications during pregnancy. They include having basic health exams, screening health tests, and vaccinations, as well as considering genetic testing, reducing occupational exposures, and dealing with any ongoing health problems you have. Later in the chapter, I provide a summary checklist for each of you to complete.

SCREENING TESTS AND HEALTH EXAMS

If you're planning a pregnancy, it's important that you have had a recent checkup and that you're up to date on your regular health screening examinations. The idea behind preventive health care is to screen for minor problems before the dramatic hormonal changes of pregnancy turn them into major complications that are more difficult to treat.

 For Both of You

If you haven't had the following exams and screening tests within the past year, make an appointment to have these exams performed.

CARDIOVASCULAR. Having a healthy heart, lungs, and circulatory system before you become pregnant will help your body meet the physiological demands of pregnancy. Your cardiovascular system will have to handle the increase in blood volume that occurs during pregnancy, and provide your developing baby with enough oxygen and nutrients. For men, a healthy cardiovascular system can help improve the quality of sperm and perk up a weak libido.

> *Blood pressure* measures how much force your heart has to generate to circulate blood through your arteries, veins, and capillaries. The increase in blood volume during pregnancy can make blood pressure rise slightly, so it's important to get high blood pressure (hypertension) under control. About 10 percent of reproductive-age women have hypertension, though most are not aware of it because it generally doesn't create symptoms until you're pregnant. Your doctor will check your blood pressure during a physical (blood pressure can rise during an examination because of nervousness, so try to relax beforehand or have it checked several different times). If it's above 130/90, request a more thorough evaluation and recommendations for lowering it. Avoid ACE inhibitors, the popular blood pressure drugs, which should not be taken while trying to conceive.

Category	Blood Pressure
Normal	120/80
Prehypertension	120/80 to 140/90
Hypertension	Above 140/90

Pulse. Your resting heart rate is the simplest way to measure your cardiovascular health. To determine your RHR, measure your pulse for 60 seconds before you get out of bed in the morning. Having a slow resting heart rate generally indicates that your heart is working efficiently and can easily accommodate the physical demands of pregnancy. Ideally, the resting heart rate for you and your partner should be below 90 beats per minute and very regular. If it's higher, discuss with your health care provider whether your pulse rate is a concern.

Cardiac evaluation. Some people may need more of a cardiac workup, depending on the findings of a general physical or their medical and family history. If you have been a regular tobacco user, for example, you should have a more thorough evaluation.

Cholesterol/triglyceride screening. This is a routine part of any physical. Too much *cholesterol,* the fatty substance that can build up in the walls of arteries, can compromise blood flow to your heart and brain, as well as to the developing baby once you're pregnant. For men, high cholesterol can also lead to erectile dysfunction. *Triglycerides,* the body's main form of stored fat, can clog arteries and worsen insulin resistance. If cholesterol or triglycerides are high, it's probably due to an abnormally high level of insulin, the rest-and-digest hormone that normally moves blood sugar out of the blood and into cells for use as energy or fat storage. Talk to your doctor about whether you have *metabolic syndrome,* a cluster of abnormalities including elevated cholesterol, high triglycerides, abdominal weight gain, and high blood pressure, all triggered by abnormally high insulin.

Complete blood count (CBC). This screening test measures the oxygen-carrying capacity of blood cells and takes a snapshot of your immune functioning and your blood-clotting abilities. The CBC diagnoses anemia, a condition in which your blood can't deliver enough oxygen to your body. Anemia occurs in about one in five reproductive-age women and may affect your fertility and the health of your pregnancy. The most common form of anemia is due to inadequate iron intake, which is easily reversible.

INSULIN RESISTANCE. In at least one out of every three couples I see for fertility issues, the man, the woman, or both have insulin resistance.

Yet it is a vastly underdiagnosed problem, partly because many health care providers are still not that familiar with it, and because of misconceptions about who is at risk. Though it's often associated with being overweight, not all people with insulin resistance have a weight problem. Some ethnic groups, such as Asian Indians, Native Americans, African Americans and others, have a high incidence of insulin resistance—20 percent or higher—in those who are of a normal weight.

Think of insulin as a hormone that promotes energy storage. Following a meal, carbohydrates are broken down into the simple sugar, glucose, which then enters your bloodstream. Your pancreas releases insulin to help shuttle the glucose into muscles, fat, the liver, and other cells of your body to be used as energy or stockpiled for later use. When you eat a high-sugar diet or one loaded with simple carbohydrates, like white flour, the food rapidly breaks down and floods your bloodstream with glucose. In response, your pancreas releases a similar surge of insulin to deal with the high amounts of glucose as fast as possible. If you continually eat this type of food, your insulin levels will consistently be elevated. Over time, muscle, liver, and fat cells become desensitized or "resistant" to insulin—just as you tune out the fragrance of a perfume you've been wearing for several hours. Eventually, more insulin is needed to do the job, until you get to the point that your pancreas can't produce enough insulin to keep up with the demand, resulting in an elevation of blood sugar and an increased risk of developing diabetes. Your risk of developing insulin resistance depends on your ethnic background, if you're sedentary, and your level of exposure to BioMutagens.

High insulin levels also affect the balance of reproductive hormones and can lead to reduced fertility. In women, it can raise levels of testosterone, and compromise egg quality. Insulin also upsets the ratio between your egg-promoting hormones, follicle-stimulating hormone (FSH) and luteinizing hormone (LH), disrupting the development of your eggs. In men, insulin stimulates fat cells to raise estrogen levels, which may lower sperm count. I recommend that you take the questionnaire on the following page to estimate your risk of insulin resistance.

DENTAL EXAM. If you haven't had a cleaning and checkup within the past year, you should get one before you try to become pregnant. Problems like chronic inflammation of the gums can dramatically increase

INSULIN RESISTANCE RISK QUESTIONNAIRE

Circle the number for each question that applies to you and then add up your risk. Men should skip questions 8, 18, 20, 21, 25, and 26. Do you have:

1. Waist circumference greater than or equal to 35 inches (greater than or equal to 40 inches for men) — 4
2. Type 2 diabetes — 4
3. High blood pressure — 3
4. High cholesterol (LDL) or high triglycerides — 3
5. Dark patches of skin on your neck, groin, or under arms or other skin folds — 3
6. Excessive weight gain — 3
7. Difficulty keeping weight off — 3
8. History of gestational diabetes — 3
9. History of delivering a baby weighing more than 9 pounds — 2
10. Family history of type 2 diabetes — 2
11. Family history of heart disease — 2
12. History of depression — 2
13. History of bipolar mood disorder — 2
14. History of anxiety — 2
15. Personal or family history of schizophrenia — 2
16. Epilepsy — 2
17. History of infertility — 2
18. History of recurrent miscarriage — 2
19. Your birth weight was less than 6 lbs or greater than 10 lbs — 2
20. Eight or fewer menstrual cycles per year — 1
21. Absent menstrual cycles for four or more consecutive months — 1
22. Rapid or irregular pulse — 1
23. Skin tags — 1
24. Extreme fatigue, hunger, or confusion 2–3 hours after a meal — 1
25. Excessive facial hair — 1
26. Thinning hair or excessive hair loss on your head — 1
27. Migraine headaches — 1
28. Hypothyroidism — 1
29. Hypoglycemia — 1

TOTAL: _____

Total your score. Here's the bottom line:

3 or less: You have a low risk of insulin resistance. Maintain your healthy lifestyle.

4 to 6: You are at high risk for insulin resistance. I recommend that you request the following tests from your health care provider: fasting serum glucose level, fasting insulin level, and glycosylated hemoglobin test (also called hemoglobin A1C) to see if you need treatment. Also review chapter 9 for more insights into how this may be affecting your ovaries.

7 or more: You already have insulin resistance. Refer to chapter 9 for more information.

HIGH PROLACTIN

Less than 0.5 percent of the population has an elevated prolactin level, but studies reveal that 17 percent of women with infertility have this hormonal imbalance, which can inhibit ovulation. Men with low libido, erectile dysfunction, or an enlarged prostate are about five times more likely to have elevated prolactin levels than those without these symptoms.

Normally, prolactin levels rise briefly in response to sexual activity or breast stimulation, such as the suckling of a newborn. But you may get chronically high levels following breast surgery, or while taking certain medications that treat psychiatric problems like schizophrenia or bipolar disorder. A far less common cause is a benign tumor in the pituitary gland called a pituitary adenoma, which accelerates the release of prolactin.

If your doctor suspects your prolactin is elevated based on your symptoms, a blood test can determine your levels. A normal prolactin level for a woman is typically less than 30 nanogram/milliliter (less than 10 ng/ml is normal for a man). This test should be repeated on a different day if your level is abnormal to confirm that it is consistently elevated. For accuracy, testing should always be performed first thing in the morning, before exercising or having breakfast.

your risk of miscarriage or preterm birth. Men should also get regular checkups and cleanings because the bacteria in their mouth can reinfect their pregnant partners. Be sure to brush and floss regularly; you can lower your risk of miscarriage by up to 70 percent just by practicing good oral hygiene.

♀ For Her

GYNECOLOGIC SCREENING. Complete these exams annually during your reproductive years.

Pelvic exam screens for a variety of benign conditions like ovarian cysts or uterine fibroids, as well as for various infectious and precancerous conditions, such as vulvar cancer. The goal is to detect problems before they occur or when they are in their most treatable state. This should not be a painful examination, so if you do experience significant discomfort, be sure to talk about it with your health care provider to rule out any possible health issues. Don't let embarrassment keep you quiet, and consider bringing your partner, friend, or sister if it will help you talk about any concerns you have.

Pap test involves gently brushing the cervix (the canal between your vagina and uterus) with a soft instrument to collect cells. The Pap can detect evidence of infection, human papillomaviruses (or genital warts), or any other changes that can lead to cancers. There are about 30 types of human papillomaviruses (HPVs) that can infect a woman's reproductive organs and affect her fertility, and four of them may lead to certain cancers. A vaccine to prevent genital warts was approved in 2006 (see "First Anticancer Vaccine," page 47). Most health care providers will also perform a screening test for sexually transmitted diseases as well during a Pap smear. According to the latest ACOG guidelines, you can have less frequent Pap testing if your exam has been negative for three consecutive years and you've been with the same partner during that time.

POSITIVE HPV TEST MAY AFFECT CONCEPTION

In 2006, a study found that fertility patients who tested positive for the human papillomavirus (HPV) had a lower chance of becoming pregnant after they received a donated embryo than women who tested negative for the virus. If you have HPV, it may interfere with the ability of an embryo to implant in your womb. It's in your best interest to consider HPV treatment prior to pursuing fertility therapy. It's a good idea to have your partner tested as well to avoid being reinfected.

THYROID HORMONE TESTING. At least 3 percent of reproductive-age women without risk factors have thyroid disturbances; low thyroid hormone, or *hypothyroidism,* is about four times more common in women with infertility than in fertile women. A lack of iodide (the dietary form of iodine), can contribute to hypothyroidism.

When thyroid hormones are low, estradiol levels dip and testosterone levels rise. Luteinizing hormone, which normally triggers ovulation, gets blunted enough to prevent ovulation. But many general physicians and OBs don't test for hypothyroidism when treating their fertility patients. Fertility specialists do test for it, but some are not treating patients with borderline hypothyroidism (sometimes called

THE HORMONE PLAYERS

Thyroid hormones. Thyroxine (T4) is the predominant thyroid hormone. It travels through the bloodstream, attached to a carrier protein, but in order for it to become active, it has to free itself from the carrier and lose one of its four iodine molecules. At that point it's known as triiodothyronine, or T3. These hormones regulate the rate of your metabolism. Thyroid imbalances also have a profound impact on your reproductive hormones, affecting your fertility as well as the health of your pregnancy after you conceive.

subclinical hypothyroidism), though the latest research suggests that these patients should be treated (see page 52 for more information). Currently, the American Thyroid Association recommends that all women get screened for thyroid disturbances at age 35. I recommend all women consider having a *screening thyroid panel* done prior to conception, and that those with borderline thyroid imbalances be treated.

PERFECT BALANCE THYROID QUESTIONNAIRE

If you're uncertain whether you should request a blood test to assess your thyroid function, use this questionnaire to gauge your risk of thyroid disorders. Circle the symptoms you have.

1. Fluid retention in your hands and/or feet   Yes   No

2. Inability to lose weight   Yes   No

3. Intolerance to cold   Yes   No

4. Forgetfulness   Yes   No

5. Depression   Yes   No

6. Family history of thyroid disease   Yes   No

7. Existing autoimmune disorder   Yes   No

8. Swelling or tenderness in the neck   Yes   No

Total your score. Here's the bottom line:

If you answered yes to numbers 7 or 8, you are at high risk for an autoimmune thyroid disorder. Make an appointment with your physician for an evaluation—you may need both a basic thyroid panel and additional blood tests for thyroid antibodies.

If you answered yes to at least *three* from 1 to 6, you may be at risk for hypothyroidism. Request an evaluation of your thyroid function.

GENDER BENDER: THYROID AND FERTILITY

Men have about a 20 percent lower risk of hypothyroidism than women and the negative impact on them is much more subtle. Although sperm production is typically normal, hypothyroidism causes male testosterone levels to drop low enough to cause low libido, erectile dysfunction, or even ejaculatory delay. Ask your partner to use the Thyroid Questionnaire to determine whether he should be tested as well.

BREAST CANCER SCREENING. Some fertility centers are now requiring mammograms for women over 40 who are undergoing IVF. The centers want to be certain that their patients are free of breast cancer before they become pregnant. Because certain cancers are sensitive to estrogen, which surges during pregnancy, it's important to be up to date on your cancer screenings. Women over 40 should have an annual mammogram. As an alternative for high-risk women and others, I recommend magnetic resonance imaging (MRI), because of its ability to detect smaller lesions and differentiate benign fluid-filled cysts from potentially cancerous solid lesions. Although MRI is more costly, there is some evidence it can be performed less frequently. All reproductive-age women should perform monthly breast self-exams to monitor subtle changes in their breasts as well.

Breast self-examination. It is normal for your breasts to change in appearance, consistency, and size on different days of your cycle, so rest assured that most changes are not related to cancer. Time your exam with the end of your menstrual cycle. If your cycles are irregular,

HIV/AIDS TESTING: NOT JUST FOR "HIGH-RISK" INDIVIDUALS

The Centers for Disease Control and Prevention (CDC) recommends universal HIV testing for all women between the ages of 13 and 64. Most fertility centers require testing for women and their partners prior to treatment. An estimated 250,000 people in the United States who are HIV-positive aren't aware of their status. Through universal testing, the hope is to diagnose and begin early treatment, as well as remove the stigma associated with getting tested. So don't be put off when you and your partner are asked to undergo testing.

pick any day of the month and consistently do it the same day of the month. Your exam should include a visual examination of your breasts and nipples, as well as careful palpation. There are a variety of techniques, so talk to your health care provider about which is most appropriate for you.

Vaccinations: Are You Up to Date?

One of the greatest advances of modern medicine has been the use of dead or weakened bacteria and viruses to prevent illness. Vaccinations can prevent infection during pregnancy, and during the last month and a half of your pregnancy, antibodies to diseases you've been vaccinated against cross the placenta to provide your baby with its initial protection from infection. So talk to your doctor about the following vaccinations:

Measles, mumps, and rubella (MMR) is a live but weakened combination of viruses that most of us have been given as a child. If you can't confirm that you've received this vaccination, a simple blood test can determine whether you're immune to these viruses, which can cause birth defects if you become infected with one of them during pregnancy. This vaccine should be given at least one month prior to conception; however, no demonstrated risks of its use during pregnancy have ever been reported. Only one dose is needed.

Tetanus, diptheria, and pertussis (Tdap) is a vaccine against certain toxins produced by bacteria that can cause lockjaw and respiratory infections like whooping cough. Immunity from this vaccination is not as strong, so a booster is needed every 10 years. This is safe during pregnancy and won't affect your fertility.

Varicella (chicken pox) can be a life-threatening infection if you become ill while pregnant. If you had chicken pox as a child, you are probably still immune to the chicken pox virus. If not, get one injection at least a month before you try to become pregnant. You cannot use this vaccine while pregnant, so be sure to use contraception for one month after being vaccinated.

Influenza (flu) is recommended for anyone who will be pregnant during the peak flu season (January–March). The injectable form is safe for use during pregnancy because it is an inactivated virus that

FIRST ANTICANCER VACCINE

Over 20 million men and women in the United States are infected by the human papillomavirus (HPV). In 2006, the first vaccine to prevent a cancer was approved by the FDA. Called Gardasil, this three-injection series is designed to prevent infection with the four most common forms of HPV, including the one associated with at least 70 percent of cervical cancers. I recommend getting vaccinated, as HPV has been associated with reduced fertility. The series takes six months in total, but you can continue it even if you become pregnant. If you already have been infected with one or more of the HPV strains, you may still benefit from the vaccine by developing immunity to those strains you have not yet encountered.

cannot cause infection. If you may be pregnant, do not use the nasal spray, which contains a weakened but live form of the vaccine.

Hepatitis A (hep A) is only needed for people at risk of exposure to this infection, which can cause liver damage. Talk to your health care provider to see if you're at risk. The vaccine contains an inactivated virus, and is safe to have during pregnancy. Two shots are needed.

Hepatitis B (hep B) is recommended for all children, as well as all adults at risk of exposure, especially health care workers. It is made from a protein associated with the bloodborne virus and is safe to take during pregnancy. Three shots are needed.

♂ For Him

TESTOSTERONE TESTING. Beginning around age 30, levels of testosterone drop by about 1 to 2 percent each year. Some men may have

THE HORMONE PLAYER

Testosterone. The leading androgen, testosterone (often mistakenly referred to as the male sex hormone), is most known for its libido-enhancing properties, but it is also behind the sexual maturity of boys and girls, helps build muscle and improve athletic performance, and is linked to self-confidence, motivation, and vigor. Testosterone also circulates in women, in whom it serves the same functions but occurs at much lower levels.

ANDROGEN DEFICIENCY SYNDROME QUESTIONNAIRE*

Answer the questions below. Take this test first thing in the morning.

1. Have you experienced a decreased libido (sex drive)? Yes No

2. Do you feel fatigue or decreased energy level? Yes No

3. Have you noticed a reduction in your strength and/or endurance? Yes No

4. Has your height decreased? Yes No

5. Have you experienced a decreased sense of wellness? Yes No

6. Are you sad, depressed, or irritable? Yes No

7. Do you have difficulty getting or maintaining an erection? Yes No

8. Has your motivation or self-confidence diminished? Yes No

9. Do you find you're falling asleep after meals or at midday? Yes No

10. Has your performance at work diminished? Yes No

Total your score. Here's the bottom line:

If you answered yes to questions 1 or 7, or to at least three of the other questions, your symptoms may be due to low testosterone. Request a blood test for total and free testosterone levels. To find a health care provider who is qualified to assess this disorder, visit www.menshealthnetwork.org.

*Modified from Androgen Deficiency in Aging (ADAM) Questionnaire developed by John Morley, M.D., at Saint Louis University, 1977.

---

symptoms such as fatigue, loss of libido, weight gain, or depression, whereas others never develop any symptoms. It's estimated that between 4 and 5 million men experience symptoms of low testosterone but that only about 5 percent ever seek treatment. When testosterone drops low enough to create these symptoms, it's referred to as *androgen deficiency syndrome,* a disorder that was recently recognized by the American Association of Clinical Endocrinologists. Hormone testing can help diagnose and correct early shifts in testosterone that could develop into long-term problems, affecting quality of life and fertility. If you think you have symptoms related to low testosterone, then take the questionnaire above and consider making an appointment with an endocrinologist to discuss your results.

PRECONCEPTION CHECKLIST

For Her			For Him		
TEST		**RESULT**	**TEST**		**RESULT**
Cardiovascular	BP (avg)	_____	Cardiovascular	BP (avg)	_____
	Pulse	_____		Pulse	_____
Cholesterol	LDL	_____	Cholesterol	LDL	_____
	HDL	_____		HDL	_____
	Total chol	_____		Total chol	_____
	Triglycerides	_____		Triglycerides	_____
CBC	Normal	_____	CBC	Normal	_____
	Anemic	_____			
Metabolic testing (fasting)	Insulin	_____	Metabolic testing (fasting)	Insulin	_____
	Glucose	_____		Glucose	_____
	HgA1c	_____		HgA1c	_____
Thyroid screening	TSH	_____	Thyroid screening	TSH	_____
	T4 free	_____		T4 free	_____
	T4 direct	_____		T4 direct	_____
	T3	_____		T3	_____
Genetic testing	_____		Genetic testing	_____	
			Androgen deficiency testing	Total T	_____
				Free T	_____

VACCINATION	DATE	RESULT	VACCINATION	DATE	RESULT
Hepatitis A	_____	_____	Hepatitis A	_____	_____
Hepatitis B	_____	_____	Hepatitis B	_____	_____
HIV screen	_____	_____	HIV screen	_____	_____

(continued)

PRECONCEPTION CHECKLIST

For Her

VACCINATION	DATE	RESULT
RPR	_____	_____
MMR	_____	_____
Tdap	_____	_____
Varicella (chicken pox)	_____	_____
Flu	_____	_____
HPV vaccine	_____	_____

EXAM	RESULT
Dental exam	_____
Pelvic exam	_____
Pap smear	_____
Breast cancer screening (BSE or mammogram if over 40)	_____

For Him

VACCINATION	DATE	RESULT
RPR	_____	_____

EXAM	RESULT
Dental exam	_____
Testicular self-exam	_____

Do breast self-exam or testicular self-exam monthly.

CANCER SCREENING. This is part of any routine physical examination and should be ordered by your doctor based upon your age and your known risk factors. You should also begin performing testicular self-examination. Testicular cancer is the most common cancer in men between puberty and age 40, affecting about 1 in every 250 reproductive-age males. This test will take you less than five minutes and should be performed once a month.

Testicular self-examination. Do this at the end of a shower. Use one hand to gently grasp your testicle between your thumb and index finger while you slowly roll your other thumb and index finger over the entire surface using gentle pressure. Note if you feel any hardened or sandy regions or if you feel any painless lumps. You'll note the *epididymis,* an elongated structure along the length of the back of each testicle. This structure normally stores and transports sperm. It is normal for one testicle to be larger than the other. Discuss any abnormalities or changes with your doctor.

CONTRACEPTION: WHEN TO STOP

Misconceptions abound regarding when to stop contraception before trying to become pregnant. Many women believe, for example, that they need to be off the pill for six months before trying to conceive. This strategy not only wastes time, but for some women, like those with polycystic ovarian syndrome (PCOS), or anorexia, it may reduce their chance of getting pregnant.

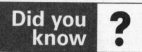

Did you know ?

Many women are most fertile in the first three months after stopping the birth control pill.

These women may miss their most fertile time—the first few cycles after stopping the pill. With the majority of hormonal contraceptives, you should stop one to two months before trying to get pregnant (see the following chart). Based upon my experience with patients, here's a quick rundown of when to discontinue different methods of contraception in relation to when your peak fertility returns—with or without treatment.

Method	May Use Until . . .
Birth control pill	
Monthly cycle	one month before desired fertility
Extended cycle	two months before desired fertility
Contraceptive patch	one to two months before desired fertility
Contraceptive vaginal ring	one month before desired fertility
Intrauterine device (IUD)	two months before desired fertility
Contraceptive implant	two months before desired fertility
Contraceptive injection	nine months before desired fertility

YOUR HISTORY OF CONTRACEPTION AND FERTILITY

You may not need contraception now, but if you used barrier contraception in the past, it helped prevent infections like chlamydia and gonorrhea that can damage your fallopian tubes and can increase your risk for more serious diseases, such as hepatitis and AIDS. It also lowers your risk of genital warts. If you didn't use barrier contraception in the past, be sure to get checked for these diseases.

MANAGING CHRONIC CONDITIONS

As more couples are waiting until their late reproductive years to become pregnant, more parents-to-be have underlying health conditions. If you have a disorder, it's critical that it's well managed before you try to conceive, as pregnancy can exacerbate some health issues. Ask your health care provider if there are medications that are safer for the developing fetus than what you're currently taking. Here are a few issues that relate to some of the most common disorders of reproductive age women.

HYPOTHYROIDISM. Treatment of low thyroid usually consists of taking a BioIdentical thyroid replacement called thyroxine. Prior to getting

---

MEDICATIONS, SUPPLEMENTS, AND HERBS

Any medication, supplement, or herb that can improve your health can also create side effects. Some can also increase risk to you or your child once you become pregnant. Talk to your doctor about the safety and dose of any medication you're taking, and make sure it won't interfere with conception and pregnancy. You should use the lowest effective dose or shift to a drug that has been shown to be safe in studies of a large group of pregnant women. I recommend considering three simple questions as they pertain to each prescription or over-the-counter medication, as well as any supplements or herbs that you or your partner are taking:

1. Why am I taking this?
2. Do I need to continue taking this?
3. Is there a safer alternative or can I safely lower my dose?

CORRECTING HYPOTHYROIDISM WITH BIOIDENTICAL HORMONES

If you and your doctor decide you'd rather use a T4-T3 combination, I recommend avoiding the "natural" Armour Thyroid, a prescription that's made from the thyroid glands of factory-farmed pigs. The problem is, the amount of thyroid hormone from one animal to the next varies, leading to inconsistency between doses. In 2005, the FDA recalled nearly 60,000 bottles of Armour Thyroid tablets due to "sub-potency." Instead, I recommend Thyrolar as a safer, synthetic BioIdentical hormone preparation.

pregnant, make sure your dose of thyroid replacement hormone is appropriate. It's best for thyroid hormone levels to be in the high end of the normal range in order to reduce your risk of miscarriage or developmental problems for your baby. Some people respond best to a combination of T4, the circulating form of thyroid, and T3, the active form. If you don't feel your best on a T4-only preparation, then talk to your doctor about adding Cytomel (the BioIdentical form of T3) or Thyrolar (a fixed-ratio combination of T4 and T3).

DIABETES. This occurs when your insulin levels are too low to keep blood sugar within a normal range. In type 1 diabetes, the pancreas fails to produce insulin, so women need to inject the BioIdentical form of this hormone several times a day. Type 2 diabetes is a combination of insulin resistance and insulin deficiency, meaning that the pancreas is producing insulin but not at sufficient levels to control blood sugar. It is essential that blood-sugar management is stabilized at least three months before conception. Doing so can dramatically reduce your risk of miscarriage and pregnancy complications, while also lowering your child's risk of birth defects. You can control blood sugar through a careful coordination of diet and exercise, which helps minimize your insulin needs (see chapter 4 on nutrition guidelines).

HYPERTENSION. In many women, an imbalance of the hormone *angiotensin* is a major cause of high blood pressure. But the popular medications called ACE inhibitors, which target angiotensin, are not safe to use while trying to conceive. Ask your doctor about changing your medication to one that's safe to use during pregnancy.

PREGNANCY FOLLOWING GASTRIC BYPASS

Surgical treatment for obesity is growing in popularity. By now, several thousand women have become pregnant following gastric bypass surgery, which reduces the capacity of the stomach and decreases the ability of the intestines to absorb calories. The evidence shows that pregnancy is safe, but should be delayed at least three to six months after surgery to allow your body to adjust to your new hormonal balance. I recommend waiting at least a year from the date of surgery. Women who have the surgery achieve a healthier state of hormone balance, including lower insulin resistance, reduced hormones that promote appetite, and improvements in the function of thyroid hormone. With this new balance comes improved fertility. This surgery is not without risk and should only be undertaken when absolutely necessary. When you do become pregnant, your care will include ensuring that you get adequate amounts of certain micronutrients (especially, iron, calcium, folic acid, and vitamin B_{12}) to support the growing baby, but you can effectively continue to lose weight—especially in the first trimester. If you've had gastric bypass or are considering it, preconception counseling is essential and should include visits with a registered dietician to ensure your safety and that of your baby.

EPILEPSY, BIPOLAR DISORDER, MIGRAINE HEADACHES, OR CHRONIC PAIN. In addition to using seizure medications to treat epilepsy, doctors are frequently prescribing these drugs to manage bipolar disorder, migraines, and chronic pain. These medications have been associated with a variety of birth defects and should be used in the lowest effective dose possible. Even many of the newer antiepilepsy drugs, like lamotrigine, which were originally touted as safer, are now known to carry some risk. Talk to your doctor about lowering your dosage of any of these medications, or ask if you might be able to wean off the medication for your first trimester, when the risk to the baby is greatest. If not, you can request switching to an extended-release preparation, which is taken fewer times each day to minimize the dose.

GENETIC TESTING: DETERMINING YOUR CHILD'S RISKS

We each carry our family health history in every cell of our body in the form of 23 pairs of chromosomes. These chromosomes constitute your genetic blueprint, directing each cell in its specific task by activating certain segments, or genes, while keeping others quiescent. In some cases, the genes you and your partner pass down may be linked to inherited diseases. You might want to consider genetic testing to predict your risk of having a child with an inheritable disease.

Below are the most common inheritable disorders you can test for, but first talk to your health care provider or a genetic counselor about how useful any test would be based on the following aspects of your personal and family history.

1. Which ethnic or racial group do you and your partner most closely identify with?
2. What is the geographic origin of you and your partner?
3. Have you previously had a child with a birth defect or inherited disorder?
4. Have you had more than one miscarriage?
5. Were you or your partner exposed to any known toxins?
6. Does anyone in your family have a history of hemophilia or any other inherited disorder?
7. Has anyone in your family had a child with mental retardation?

Common Inheritable Disorders

Cystic fibrosis, a severe disease of the lungs, affects about 1 in 3,300 Americans, but many more people carry a gene defect that can cause it. Your child can only develop it if both you and your partner are carriers. If you're Caucasian, the chance that you or your partner is a carrier can be as high as 1 in 25; if you're Hispanic, it's 1 in 46; African American, it's 1 in 65; and Asian, it's 1 in 90. Since this condition is life-threatening, testing is offered to all reproductive age couples planning pregnancy.

Tay-Sachs disease results in severe disabilities related to the nervous system. If you're of Ashkanazi (Eastern European) Jewish, French Canadian, Pennsylvania Dutch, or southern Cajun descent, you are at higher risk.

Fragile X syndrome is the most common inherited cause of mental retardation, occurring in about 1 of 4,000 male infants born and 1 of

8,000 females. Since about 1 in 260 women are carriers, I recommend testing. If you test positive, your child has about a 50 percent chance of developing this disorder. If you have a family history of premature onset of menopause, you may be at a higher than average risk for passing down fragile X, so testing is recommended.

MATERNAL AGE AND RISK OF INHERITED DISEASE

As women age, more of their eggs develop genetic changes. This raises the risk of having a baby with chromosomal problems. Most of these pregnancies miscarry early in the first trimester and the overall risk may be lower than you would assume. There are prenatal tests available once you become pregnant to screen for many of these inherited problems.

Age-Related Risk of Delivering an Infant with a Chromosomal Abnormality

Maternal Age at Delivery	Affected Infants per 1,000 Live Births
20	2
25	2
30	3
35	5
40	15
45	48

INHERITED ANEMIAS: NONGENETIC SCREENING TESTS

There are several inherited forms of anemia, in which your blood can't carry enough oxygen throughout your body. It can be caused by red blood cells that are unusually fragile or that have a shortened life span. A blood test that examines blood cells, not genes, can determine whether cells are abnormally shaped and smaller than normal. The type of anemia is then confirmed through another kind of blood test. Below are the most common inherited forms of anemia and the groups at highest risk. If your or your partner's family comes from one of these regions or if you have a family history of these or other blood disorders, talk to your doctor about testing to see if you're a carrier.

Inherited Disorder	People at Highest Risk From . . .
Sickle-cell anemia	Africa
Alpha-thalassemia	China and Southeast Asia
Beta-thalassemia	Mediterranean

◆　　◆　　◆

Many of the healthful changes that you make during the next several months will improve your fertility rate as well as your child's health. Remember that it takes many months for an egg to mature and about three months for sperm to fully mature. So start your preconception plan and use the next few months to implement the nutrition, exercise, and mind-body programs that follow, and you may find that you won't need fertility treatments at all.

4 Eating Right for Fertility

Food has always been intimately linked to our ability to reproduce. A quick look back to primitive times provides evidence of how our bodies function and reproduce most naturally. The fertility rates of our hunter-gatherer ancestors ebbed and flowed with the availability of food. A bountiful fall harvest would result in a springtime boon in deliveries. During times of drought and famine, fertility rates would drop—a natural protection against malnourished pregnancies. In these extreme circumstances, the brain's nutritional sensor would literally turn off the hormonal signals to ovulate, a response that still lingers in our society today as witnessed in people with anorexia, who starve themselves. But history doesn't provide us any insight on the opposite condition—the impact of an overabundance of food on fertility. In today's world of sustained food production, we are learning that calorie excess can be just as, if not more, harmful to fertility as food deprivation. It causes its own set of hormone imbalances that shut off the brain's fertility signals. So, too, does the type of food we eat—processed high-sugar, high-fat foods—and the food we don't eat enough of—fruits, vegetables, and fiber. Fortunately, the artificial and unhealthy diet we have created can easily be corrected.

About 65 percent of Americans are overweight or obese. If you are in this group, losing weight is your first step toward improving your fertility. But your daily calorie balance is equally, if not more important, than

Case in Point

When I first met Maureen and Alan, they had been trying to conceive for nearly three years. They were scared, because Alan's parents took nearly 12 years to conceive him, and they had quickly drawn parallels to their own lives. After a basic evaluation, we established that Maureen, 27, was ovulating each month and did not have any signs of fertility problems. Alan, though, at 36, had a very low sperm count and low motility (his sperm moved sluggishly). Alan was very overweight and I had suspected that he had insulin resistance, which in men can lower sperm count and function. I suggested that we focus on boosting his fertility by improving his hormone balance.

My nutritionist recommended healthier food choices, focusing on increasing his fiber and moderately reducing his calories. I also recommended he take an over-the-counter supplement called ConceptionXR, containing nutrients that improve sperm health. I encouraged them to begin eating organic food to lower his exposure to processed unhealthy foods that were contributing to his hormone imbalance. We scheduled a follow-up semen analysis in three months and agreed to check in at six months to consider fertility treatments if they had not conceived by then. After four months, Maureen announced her pregnancy. When they came in for their first ultrasound, Alan had lost 28 pounds and was feeling better than he ever had. Maureen delivered a healthy baby girl.

how much weight you lose. In other words, simply not overeating on a daily basis will improve your fertility long before you reach your ideal body weight.

At the other end of the weight spectrum, women and men that are severely underweight also become less fertile—ovulation stops in women and sperm production drops in men. Very thin women, even if

GENDER BENDER: OBESITY'S AFFECT ON TESTOSTERONE

When a woman becomes obese, her hypothalamus signals her ovaries to create a rise in testosterone, which interrupts ovulation. When a man packs on the pounds, his testosterone levels drop, causing erectile dysfunction and low libido. About half of obese men experience sexual dysfunction that may prohibit intercourse.

they are still ovulating, are also at risk of a fertilized egg not implanting. Studies suggest that about 6 percent of reproductive-age women have an eating disorder such as anorexia, bulimia, or binge-eating disorder (see "Eating Disorders and Infertility," page 68). In my practice, nearly 20 percent of the women I see with infertility have an eating disorder. Whether you're too thin or overweight, restoring hormone balance by making better food choices can dramatically improve your success rate in as little as six weeks.

Case in Point

When Vanessa, 24, and Ryan, 31, came to see me, they had been trying to get pregnant for nearly four years and had already gone through several failed treatment attempts with another specialist. We began our first visit by reviewing all their previous tests and treatments. They had expected me to recommend a more high-tech and expensive treatment, but instead I suggested they consider their diet. Vanessa's eyebrows raised and she began to squirm with discomfort.

I gently suggested that at five feet four inches and 95 pounds, she was very thin for her frame. She confided her long history of anorexia, but felt like she had her problem under control. I explained that at her current weight, she did not have enough calories stored to sustain a healthy pregnancy. Vanessa eventually agreed to set a goal of 110 pounds before we considered any further treatments. She met with my nutritionist to develop a healthy plan to gain weight gradually. I also recommended she begin taking a prenatal vitamin and shift to organic foods. It took continued encouragement and coaching from her husband, but Vanessa slowly began to ease her personal restrictions and gain weight. When she reached 102 pounds, her menstrual cycles became regular for the first time in eight years. When she hit 108 pounds, about three months after our initial visit, she conceived—without any treatment. She continued to see the nutritionist throughout her pregnancy to make sure that she gained weight appropriately as her pregnancy progressed, and delivered a healthy baby girl.

WEIGHT-FERTILITY CONNECTION

Your hormones determine what your body does with the calories you eat. Are they going to be used immediately as fuel by your brain, stored in your muscles and liver for short-term use, or deposited in fat

THE MOST COMMON HORMONAL CAUSE OF INFERTILITY

The most common hormonal disorder of reproductive age women and the leading hormonal cause of infertility is polycystic ovarian syndrome (PCOS), a hormonal imbalance of high insulin and testosterone levels, often resulting in symptoms like weight gain, acne, and menstrual irregularity (for more information, see chapter 9). PCOS is frequently treated with birth control pills to regulate menstrual cycles and reduce other symptoms. But this approach has given health care providers a false sense that they are treating this condition. Instead, they are simply masking its symptoms. Several years ago, a panel of PCOS experts concluded that treatment of these patients should be directed toward treating its underlying cause, insulin resistance, by improving the body's sensitivity to insulin. The best ways to accomplish this is through better diet.

cells as a long-term energy supply? Researchers are continually discovering new hormones that play a role in weight gain and loss, but insulin is the main player. If you consume too many calories at once or choose foods that are absorbed too rapidly, your insulin can't shuttle glucose into muscle and liver cells efficiently. Instead, it gets stored as fat—in as little as two hours—leading to weight gain, and setting you up for insulin resistance and diabetes along with reduced fertility. If, on the other hand, you don't eat enough, you won't store enough glucose in your liver. Your liver is responsible for releasing glucose back into the bloodstream between meals and throughout the night. Here lies an important link to fertility. In the middle of the night, your brain sends signals to your ovary to ovulate, but if your brain senses low

Fertility Fact

The Obesity Dilemma

Over the last 25 years, infertility rates have risen in proportion to the rise in obesity in men and women in their reproductive years. One analysis determined that at least 10 percent of today's fertility problems are related to overeating. The good news for obese people is that losing 10 percent of your body weight will improve your chance of conception (if you're overweight, not obese, you'll see the benefits after losing only 5 percent of your body weight). So create short-term goals on your path to hormone balance and don't focus on attaining your ideal body weight.

glucose levels at night, it interprets this as a shortage of energy reserves. Your brain thinks that you don't have the calories to sustain a pregnancy—and you very well may not—and therefore won't release the hormonal signal to ovulate. Eating right can help these hormones stay in balance and restore your fertility.

EATING RIGHT FOR PERFECT BALANCE

Don't think of this as a diet, but rather as a nutrition makeover. I'll provide you with a list of principles that encourage healthier food choices and improve your satisfaction after meals, without creating any sense of deprivation. Studies show that restrictive dieting encourages cravings, weight gain, and poor nutrition. Instead, this plan allows you to feel satisfied without triggering hormonal chaos. The foundation of my plan is to reduce the amount of processed foods you eat, and replace them with fresh, whole-food alternatives. These foods are those in their most natural form, like fresh fruits and vegetables, nuts, and whole grains. They're packed with fiber and other nutrients that keep your hormones balanced and your hunger sated. Processed foods, on the other hand, tend to have many of their nutrients processed out of them. Processed foods can also trigger hormone imbalances and encourage overeating because they don't satisfy your hunger.

PRINCIPLE ONE: YOUR ENERGY NEEDS FOR FERTILITY

Now that we've established that being too thin or too fat can lead to infertility, it's important to try to achieve a healthy weight. The best way to do this is to know your individual calorie needs—most people overestimate how many calories they need in a day, leading to weight gain. Follow this three-step process to determine if you'll need to decrease or increase your calorie intake, or stay just as you are, to achieve perfect balance.

Step 1: Determine Your BMI

Knowing your *body mass index (BMI),* a rough estimate of your fat stores, gives you a basic idea of whether you need to lose or gain weight or stay the same for optimum fertility. But don't be daunted: if you adjust your diet, your hormone balance will shift to a healthier state long before you reach the Perfect Balance Fertility Zone.

First, determine your BMI using this equation: your weight (in pounds) ÷ (your height in inches × height in inches) × 703 = **BMI**_____. (For example: 130 lbs ÷ (66″ × 66″) × 703 = BMI 20.) Then see where you fall on the chart below to determine whether you need to lose, gain, or stay the same to be in the Perfect Balance Fertility Zone.

BMI	Weight Status
Below 18.5	Underweight
18.5–24.9	Perfect Balance Fertility Zone
25.0–29.9	Overweight
30.0 and Above	Obese

Step 2: Calculate Your BMR

Since we all have different energy needs depending on our activity level, our size, our age, and our environment, you need to probe a bit deeper to figure out your daily calorie needs. For example, BMI does not take into account whether a person has fat or muscle mass (muscle weighs more), so a very-well-conditioned, muscular athlete might be inaccurately classified as obese.

Your *basal metabolic rate (BMR)* is the rate at which you burn calories while at rest. Your BMR accounts for approximately 60 to 75 percent of the calories you burn each day just to stay alive. You need to know this to figure out what your individual calorie intake should be. To calculate your BMR:*

Number

1. Multiply your weight in pounds by 4.3: _____

2. Multiply your height in inches by 4.7: _____

3. Multiply your age in years by 4.7: _____

4. Add the numbers from #1 and #2, then subtract #3: _____

5. Now add 655 to #4: **YOUR BMR:** _____

*Harris Benedict Formula

Step 3: Input Your Activity Level

Now factor in your activity level to determine how many calories you are burning per day. Select the category you fall into, and multiply your BMR by the number shown.

Sedentary (desk job, little or no exercise)	BMR x 1.2
Light activity (light exercise 1 to 3 days/week)	BMR x 1.375
Moderate activity (moderate exercise 3 to 5 days/week)	BMR x 1.55
Very active (6–7 day/week)	BMR x 1.725
Extreme (hard every day, endurance training)	BMR x 1.9

TOTAL CALORIES BURNED PER DAY _____

Putting It All Together

Your total calories burned per day is the same amount of calories you need to consume to *maintain* your current weight. If you need to *lose* weight, based on your BMI, eat about 250 to 300 fewer calories per day than your total calories burned, and increase your exercise so you're burning 250 calories more per day, for a total of a 500-calorie daily deficit (see chapter 5 on exercising calories away). If you need to *gain* weight, consume 500 calories more each day (of healthy food). With each approach, you'll gain or lose about 1 to 2 pounds per week. That's a healthy rate of weight change and will promote your efforts to conceive. If you try to lose too rapidly, you'll create a hormone imbalance that will reduce your chance of producing healthy eggs or sperm and lose some muscle as well. If you gain too rapidly by consuming too many calories—or too many unhealthy calories—you'll trigger hormonal imbalance and increase the production of damaging free radicals.

Perfect Balance Alternatives to Trim Calories

It is easier to lose weight without feeling deprived if you trim 50 to 100 calories here and there from your diet rather than skip meals or snacks completely or eliminate groups of foods you really like. Consider the following list as examples of how to swap high-calorie foods for lower-calorie, healthier alternatives. When considering low-calorie

Fertility Fact

Free Radicals Affect Fertility

Eating fewer calories has the added benefit of lowering your production of *free radicals*—small charged (oxidized) particles that are produced as you digest food. Oxygen is used in the breakdown of food, and as the oxygen is metabolized, it creates free radicals as a by-product. Free radicals can damage proteins, cell membranes, and even the DNA in your eggs and your partner's sperm. The damage occurs when free radicals attach to healthy cells and release their charge. The more calories you consume, the more free radicals you produce. When you eat too many calories, your body's supply of antioxidants (which normally protect against free radicals by absorbing their charge) can't keep up with the glut of free radicals. As you reduce your calories, you have fewer free radicals causing havoc.

Sperm are particularly susceptible to free radicals. While free radical damage that occurs in most cells is repaired, sperm lack the ability to mend the damage. Severely damaged sperm may lose their ability to swim toward your egg or even acquire genetic defects. In women, free radicals can damage the DNA in eggs and the vital structures that help the egg reach maturity. The cumulative effect of years of free radical damage contributes to the age-related increase in miscarriage and birth defects. It is important for both you and your partner to avoid overeating to reduce exposure to free radicals.

food substitutions, be aware that many "lite" foods contain unhealthy amounts of sodium or sugar and often contain ingredients that may make the food less nutritious, such as preservatives, additives, or chemicals.

INSTEAD OF:	SWITCH TO:	CALORIES SAVED
1 tbsp butter for cooking	Olive oil cooking spray	75
1½ cups cold cereal	1 cup	50
8 oz orange juice	1 medium orange	35
Using half-and-half in your coffee	2% milk	50
Commercially sweetened iced tea	Carbonated water—plain or flavored but unsweetened	90 (per 8 oz)
12 oz soda	Diet soda	150

INSTEAD OF:	SWITCH TO:	CALORIES SAVED
Cream-based soup	Broth-based soup	100–200
A traditional sandwich	An open-faced sandwich	70–120
1 tbsp mayonnaise on a sandwich or wrap	1 tbsp mustard	90
2 tbsp cream-based salad dressing	2 tbsp vinaigrette	100
¼ cup pesto sauce	½ cup marinara	80–160
1 cup brown rice	½ cup brown rice	110
Softening vegetables in oil or butter	Soften in broth	90–180
3 oz ground beef—80% lean	3 oz ground beef—93% lean	90
½ cup banana chips	1 medium banana	125
½ cup ice cream	½ cup nonfat frozen yogurt	150
A slice of chocolate cake	½ slice—share with a friend	120
Breaded boneless, skinless chicken breast	Grilled boneless skinless chicken breast	160
Coffee house muffin	Biscotti	250–390
1 large bagel with light cream cheese	Whole wheat English muffin with preserves	160–200
8 oz of beef (the size of two decks of cards)	3 oz of beef (the size of a deck of cards)	225
A Burger King Whopper	Junior Whopper without mayonnaise	380
Chicken fajitas—fast food	3 chicken tacos	200

If You Need to Gain Weight, Add a Few Healthy Calories

If you are underweight or have trouble maintaining lean body mass, you might need to consume small, frequent meals and snacks every two to three hours. Increase your caloric intake slowly. An extra 100 calories per day add up to nearly one pound a month. The following healthy foods contain 125 calories or less and are a great addition to any diet.

Add	Gain (cals)
5 walnuts or almonds	125
¼ cup granola	125
4.4 oz container nonfat fruit yogurt	117
8 oz glass skim milk	100

Add	Gain (cals)
8 oz minestrone soup	125
1 whole egg, large	90
1 whole egg white, large	17
1 medium apple	72
1 cup broccoli	30
1 cup blueberries	44
1 medium banana	105
1 oz low-fat mozzarella cheese	71
1 tbsp peanut butter	94
1/2 medium avocado	112
1/4 block (2.8 oz) firm tofu	119

EATING DISORDERS AND INFERTILITY

Eating disorders can be a major obstacle to fertility. If you feel you or your partner have an eating disorder, seek a qualified health care professional before pursuing fertility treatment so that you can establish a relationship with someone who can follow up through pregnancy and delivery. Managing the disorder will improve your health and your success rate. Eating disorders fall into these three designated categories.

◆ **Anorexia nervosa** is the inability to maintain a healthy minimum body weight combined with a fear of gaining weight. Nine out of 10 people with this disorder are women. Their unusually low body fat interrupts the signal that triggers the brain to signal the ovaries to ovulate. As a result, they stop menstruating.

◆ **Bulimia nervosa** involves binge eating followed by frequent extreme measures to purge the calories, such as inducing vomiting, the abuse of laxatives, excessive exercising, or prolonged fasting. Many people with this disorder have a normal weight, but the fluctuation in calories from feast to famine triggers fat cells to send chaotic messages that can cause thyroid imbalances and disrupt the maturing of eggs and ovulation.

◆ **Eating disorder not otherwise specified** includes variations of anorexia and bulimia that don't meet the criteria of either one. Some women with anorexia may gain enough weight to menstruate but are still too thin. Some binge-and-purge eaters may not do it frequently enough to fit the bulimia criteria. This category also includes people with binge-eating disorder, defined by regularly bingeing in a two-hour period followed by a prolonged fast. These disorders can also throw your body off-kilter and have varying effects on fertility.

PRINCIPLE TWO:
TIME TO GO ORGANIC

Many of our conventionally grown food choices and beverages are loaded with pesticides, fungicides, herbicides, preservatives, additives, and antibiotics. It's estimated that about 90 percent of our total intake of these chemicals come from processed foods that we eat, and most of these ingredients are classified as *hormone disrupters.*

A hormone disrupter is any chemical that mimics a hormone, blocks a hormone receptor, or triggers a hormone imbalance by increasing hormone production or preventing its elimination. These BioMutagens have the ability to reduce fertility, promote miscarriage, or encourage the formation of cancers and other diseases. We used to simply disregard these chemicals, because they were categorized as "generally recognized as safe." Yet, over the last 10 years, research has consistently found

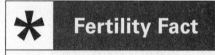

Fertility Fact

Nonorganic Dairy Products Increase Risk of Twins

A 2006 study demonstrated that women who ate two or more servings of nonorganic dairy products a day were five times as likely to have twins as women who didn't eat dairy at all. Looking for an explanation, the researchers found that the rise in twins correlated with dairy farmers' increased use of a hormone called insulin-like growth factor (IGF). Farmers regularly inject IGF into dairy cows to increase their milk output. But IGF is excreted into the milk and is passed to those who eat dairy products. Other studies in women have found that IGF stimulates the ovaries to release a larger number of eggs during ovulation. By comparison, women in Britain, where the use of IGF has been banned, are less than half as likely to have twins. To lower your chances of twins, seek out organic dairy products.

that many, if not most, of these chemicals are not safe at all. For example, commonly used pesticides in commercial farming and home gardening like *lindane* and the herbicide *atrazine* can block ovulation or prevent normal hormone formation afterward. Common fungicides can disrupt normal thyroid function and reduce sperm production.

Organic food is grown without artificial pesticides, herbicides, and fungicides, has not been treated with additives, preservatives, or ionizing radiation, and is free of any genetic manipulation. Over the past several years, the sale of organic products has increased by over 30 percent as they have become more widely available and their cost has come down.

FERTILITY FOES

If you're on a limited budget and can't buy all organic produce, consider at least buying organic versions of these fruits and vegetables, which, if conventionally grown, tend to have the highest content of BioMutagens of all fruits and vegetables.

Apples	Bell peppers	Celery
Cherries	Grapes	Nectarines
Peaches	Pears	Potatoes
Raspberries	Spinach	Strawberries

Jumping on this organic bandwagon has become much easier as large retailers like Wal-Mart and warehouse stores like Costco have joined longtime organic advocates like Whole Foods and Fresh Fields. But organic foods can still be more expensive and difficult to get than conventionally grown foods. If you're on a budget, limit your organic purchases to animal products, which contain the highest levels of BioMutagens found in foods. Additionally, reduce your consumption of shellfish and large fish like tuna and swordfish, which are high in dioxins, PCBs, and mercury. Dioxins can lower your thyroid levels and adversely affect your fertility. The most harmful BioMutagens are contained in the fat of meat and fish, so always buy lean and low-fat products. You can also prioritize your organic purchases to those foods you most frequently consume. If, for instance, you or your family drink milk every day, buy only organic, growth-hormone-free milk. If you eat an apple a day, make it organic also.

Fertility Fact

Add Hot Pepper

Repeated studies have demonstrated that eating foods with chili and other hot peppers reduces insulin resistance and promotes healthy hormone balance. Peppers contain capsaicin, a chemical that promotes metabolism and lowers insulin levels by up to 40 percent. This can also help with weight loss.

PRINCIPLE THREE: POWER CARBS

Over the last decade or so, carbohydrates have gotten a bad rap. Several no-carb diets were designed to reduce the worst contributors to obesity in our society, but they had the unintentional effect of reducing all carbohydrates—the good carbs as well as the bad carbs. The bad carbs, which I call *Chaos Carbs* because they can lead to spikes and dips in insulin and blood sugar levels, are highly processed sugars and starches. Food processing has extracted simple sugars from fruits and vegetables to make inexpensive sweeteners like *high-fructose corn syrup* to sweeten juices, soda, and sauces. These concentrated syrups are absorbed very rapidly, triggering a dramatic spike in insulin, which in turn sets off a series of hormonal changes that invite obesity, diabetes, and infertility.

THE HORMONE PLAYERS: INCRETINS

Incretins are a recently discovered group of insulin-sensitizing hormones that are produced by the stomach, the pancreas, and the intestines. They have become the target of pharmaceutical companies because they enhance the release of insulin and help stabilize blood sugar. They also play the most direct role in your food choices because their release is dependent upon when, how much, and what you eat. As you lose weight, your body starts correcting imbalances of incretins and improving your fertility. Here are the emerging players.

◆ **Ghrelin** is produced by your empty stomach to stimulate your appetite and boost the release of growth hormone from your brain. Growth hormone in turn stimulates your liver to release glucose, maintaining your energy level between meals. Ghrelin has recently been found to target the uterus, the testicles, and the developing embryo, but its exact function is not yet known.

◆ **Glucagon-like peptide-1,** released by your small intestines after you eat, makes you feel sated and helps your muscle and fat cells take in glucose. Unfortunately, this helpful hormone only circulates in your blood for a few minutes after release, limiting its effectiveness.

◆ **PYY3-36** is a key appetite-regulating hormone. Released from your intestine during digestion, it signals your brain to stop eating. Foods rich in protein and complex carbohydrates boost PYY3-36. Eating slowly allows this hormone to reduce the amount of food it will take to satisfy your appetite.

◆ **Amylin** is released by the same pancreatic cells that produce insulin. Amylin assists insulin in directing sugar into muscle and liver cells. It also helps you feel full longer, by slowing absorption of your last meal.

TURN CHAOS CARBS INTO POWER CARBS	
If You Like:	**Try This Instead:**
Applesauce	Raw apple with skin
Lite maple syrup (contains high-fructose corn syrup)	100% maple syrup
Mashed potatoes	Baked potato with skin
Processed tomato products (containing high-fructose corn syrup)	Organic products or fresh tomato
Short-grain white rice	Jasmine rice
Basmati rice	Barley
Strawberry milk shake	Low-fat berry smoothie
Fruit juice	Carbonated water
Instant hot cereal	5-minute oatmeal
French bread	9-grain or pumpernickel bread
Chocolate chip cookies	Oatmeal chocolate chip cookies with walnuts
Sweetened fruit rollups	Dried fruit pieces or leather
Deep-dish pizza	Thin-crust pizza
Baked beans	Dried, cooked beans
Cream of mushroom soup	Mushroom and barley soup
Refined pasta	Whole wheat pasta

The good carbohydrates, which I call *Power Carbs,* are the most important fuel source in your diet—you definitely don't want to avoid them. Power Carbs include simple sugars, most prevalent in fruits and vegetables. Because they are naturally in the company of fiber and water, their absorption is slow and they do not cause a spike in insulin. They also include complex sugars, such as whole-grain flour, potatoes, and brown rice. Complex sugars require digestion to break them down, providing a slow and more sustained release of sugar. On the contrary, the processed grains, like white breads, maintain little fiber, so they're digested quickly.

Power Carbs are the primary fuel for your brain and your muscles— they are the most efficient fuel because they can be digested using the least amount of water and energy and are used by your body most readily. Studies show that both intellectuals and athletes fall shy of their peak performance on a "low-carb" diet. Carbohydrates are also the most important fuel for a developing baby during a pregnancy. So choosing the right carbohydrates can actually promote hormone balance, and your fertility.

I recommend that about 40 to 50 percent of your calories come from Power Carbs; this will give you stamina, increased alertness, and less of an appetite throughout the day. It will help balance insulin, incretins, and other rest-and-digest hormones, which will in turn stabilize your fertility hormones.

PRINCIPLE FOUR: EAT MORE FIBER AND WHOLE GRAINS

One of the most hormonally disruptive aspects of our modern diet is that it is so low in fiber. Our digestive system and physiology is most comfortable with a high-fiber, plant-based diet. Yet, over the last century, most of our fiber-containing food has been "refined" by processing out the most nutritious part, the husk, leaving behind only the starchy white endosperm of grains like wheat. This robs us of the fiber and many nutrients. The answer to this trade-off has been to "enrich" flours by adding back nutrients, but fiber doesn't typically make it back in.

Fiber is the nondigestible carbohydrate within plant-based food. It comes in two forms, soluble and insoluble, both of which slow the absorption of sugars and improve digestion. They also aid in the elimination of waste, including excess hormones like estrogen and testosterone, and help to maintain balance of these hormones.

The average American eats between 5 and 15 grams of fiber per day. Yet, study after study shows that we should be consuming 30 to 40 grams per day to maintain hormone balance. By making this simple dietary shift, you can lower your insulin levels and have more energy between meals.

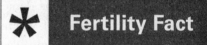

✱ Fertility Fact

Chaos Carbs Lower Libido

After you eat Chaos Carbs, the rapid sugar peak is followed by a deep lull referred to as *postprandial hypoglycemia.* The hypoglycemia, or low blood sugar, is the result of the rapid release of insulin, which also causes a drop in your testosterone. Both men and women may perceive this as a drop in their libido following a big meal. If you eat Chaos Carbs on a regular basis, this chronic drop in your testosterone level can also cause you to lose muscle mass, resulting in fatigue and decreased strength—not great for promoting sex, either. Power Carbs, by contrast, actually pack muscles with energy.

Multiple studies have demonstrated that a high-fiber diet will also help you lose weight if you're overweight or prevent weight gain if you're at a healthy weight. People who eat 40 grams of fiber per day tend to be nearly 10 pounds lighter than age-matched peers who eat the typical 8 to 10 grams per day, and they are at least 25 percent less likely to be obese. Include foods rich in fiber like these natural whole foods throughout the day.

GREAT FOODS TO BOOST DIETARY FIBER	
Soluble Fiber	**Insoluble Fiber**
Oat bran and oatmeal	Whole-grain products
Barley	Wheat bran
Rice bran	Bran flakes
Chickpeas (garbanzos)	Brown rice
Most types of beans	Pear w/skin
Lentils	Berries
Bananas	Peach w/skin
Cherries	Apple w/skin
Citrus fruit	Peas
Dried plums	Spinach
Potato	Broccoli
Sweet potato, peeled	Green beans
Black-eyed peas	Sunflower seeds
Soybeans	Almonds

You can also take fiber supplements, which contain about 5 grams of fiber per tablespoon, to improve your diet. For instance, taking a fiber supplement along with eating a piece of cake makes a Chaos Carb more like a Power Carb. This is one way you can indulge from time to time, but the spoonful of fiber trick is not license to splurge regularly—fiber can only reduce, not entirely prevent, the rapid hormonal shifts caused by processed foods. Soluble fiber supplements can easily be dissolved in any noncarbonated liquid, and they're also available in flavored tablets.

THE NEWLY DISCOVERED FAT HORMONES

Fat cells are not passive calorie warehouses, but rather mini endocrine factories that produce at least 20 different hormones, collectively called *adipokines*. These hormones direct your metabolism and help your brain keep track of your energy stores to control appetite and budget how your body uses this energy. Adipokines also help your brain determine if you have enough fat stores to sustain pregnancy. Your brain also takes into account how effectively you can share your energy with your baby—if you're insulin resistant, your body doesn't channel energy to the fetus as effectively. As you modify your diet, fat cells adjust their adipokine secretions to bring them more into balance, improving your fertility profile. Here are the key adipokines and how they affect your weight.

◆ **Leptin** tracks how many calories you have stored as fat—the more fat you have, the more leptin in your blood. When leptin levels are high, your brain suppresses your appetite and revs your metabolism to help you burn calories. But when leptin is chronically elevated, as it is in obesity, your brain tunes out the appetite-suppressing effect. Low leptin, on the other hand, signals low fat stores—a red flag that your brain should halt ovulation.

◆ **Adiponectin** helps your body use fat as fuel. As you gain weight, though, you produce less adiponectin, and low levels are associated with fertility problems. As you lose weight, fat cells release more adiponectin, increasing your chance of conception.

◆ **Resistin** is released by fat cells, *resisting* insulin's ability to help store glucose. If you're overweight, resistin rises, leading to insulin resistance and reduced fertility.

PRINCIPLE FIVE: LOW FAT IS BETTER THAN NO FAT

Before there were the unhealthy no-carb diets, there were the unhealthy no-fat diets, a diet phenomenon that led to fat-free dressings, sauces, cookies, and many more processed foods. Fats are a necessary part of your diet and play important roles in how your body functions. Aside from providing long-term energy storage, many fats serve as basic building blocks of cell membranes, insulate nerves so that they can transmit signals better, and donate carbon atoms, which your body uses to make enzymes and hormones. Fats also improve the texture and taste of our food and make us feel full, so without them, we often feel deprived of satisfying food. It's true that they pack about three times

HOW MUCH FAT?

Watching fat intake is not easy, since fat is hidden in many foods, especially processed foods. When whole foods, which have less hidden fat, make up the majority of your diet, you can safely include 3 to 5 servings per day of the following healthy fats.

Olive oil—1 tsp

Canola oil—1 tsp

Flaxseed oil—1 tsp

Flaxseed ground—1 tbsp

Nuts—2 tsp

Seeds—2 tsp

more calories per gram (12 per gram) than carbohydrates or protein, so you need to eat them in moderation. To have a balanced diet, aim for between 20 and 30 percent of your daily calorie intake coming from fats and oils.

The type of fat you eat is equally as important as how much you eat. Oils made by most plants are the healthy fats, which I call *Fluid Fats,* because they are liquid at room temperature. Most fluid fats lower unhealthy cholesterol in the blood, and a few—the monounsaturated oils, like olive oil or canola oil—also raise the good cholesterol, HDL.

The saturated fats in animal products are the unhealthy fats. They are gelatinous at room temperature, so I call these *Firm Fats.* Palm oil and coconut butter, though oils, are considered Firm Fats and should also be consumed sparingly. Firm Fats are absorbed into the bloodstream, where they contribute to artery-narrowing plaques. They also include man-made fats like trans fats, in which a hydrogen molecule is added to the fat to cause it to harden. In 2007, a study of nearly 19,000 women without a history of infertility found that when trans fats were consumed instead of healthier Fluid Fats, the women's risk of not ovulating was more than doubled. The study also found that for every 2 percent increase in calories from trans fats rather than carbohydrates, women experienced a nearly 75 percent increase in ovulatory infertility.

PRINCIPLE SIX: BECOME A FERTILE FLEXITARIAN

The amino acids that make up proteins are the building blocks of muscles, nerves, and virtually all the cells in your body. Proteins also serve as an alternate fuel source for your body. To be sure, proteins are essential, but most Americans think they need to get their protein from meat, chicken, fish, dairy products, or eggs.

Not true: Our hunter-gatherer ancestors relied heavily on plant foods, which were the most plentiful. Yet, the industrialization of food production shifted our food choices towards animal-based protein. Ultimately, we've developed a pattern of basing each meal on animal protein.

Animal products, though, contain some of the highest levels of Bio-Mutagens. Animals store hormone-disrupting chemicals in their fat tissue, where they tend to accumulate over the animal's lifetime. These chemical-fat stores can get very concentrated because most beef, pork, and poultry are raised in large factory farms that use hormone-disrupting pesticides, insecticides, herbicides, and antibiotics to reduce diseases among the animals. One study that compared protein boosts of a soy supplement to a meat supplement in women between 20 and 30

GETTING YOUR PROTEIN FROM PLANT FOODS

Here are some suggestions to modify your meals so that you can meet your protein needs from cleaner plant proteins. Choose two to three servings a day from this list. If you eat one serving of dairy, eggs, or animal protein, decrease your plant proteins to two servings per day.

Breakfast	Lunch	Dinner	Snacks
Oatmeal	Whole wheat pasta	Brown rice	Hummus
Whole wheat cereal	9-grain bread	Lentils	Peanut butter
Whole-grain bagel	3-bean salad	Pinto beans	Almonds
Low-fat granola	Split peas	Tofu or seitan	Edamame
Soy milk	Whole wheat pita	Texturized vegetable protein	Soy cheese

Fertility Fact

The Cholesterol Paradox

Although cholesterol is associated with heart disease, you couldn't live without it. Cholesterol is the basic building block for a large variety of vital hormones. Normally, about 80 percent of your cholesterol is produced by your own body, primarily by your liver. But many of us exceed our cholesterol needs when we base our diet on meat and dairy. By adopting a Flexitarian diet, you'll naturally lower your cholesterol intake and reduce your risk of heart disease while improving your fertility.

years of age found that the soy improved their hormone balance by normalizing the release of the egg-promoting hormones (FSH and LH), whereas the meat created an imbalance in these hormones that could hamper the maturation of eggs and prevent ovulation.

I appreciate that most people enjoy meat, fish, poultry, and dairy products, and might not want to eliminate them completely from their diet. Instead, I suggest you begin thinking of them as a complement to your meals rather than serving them as the main course. That's the basis of being a *Flexitarian,* or a flexible vegetarian. By reducing the amount of animal-based food you consume, you'll lower this key trigger of hormone imbalance. I recommend that 30 to 40 percent of your daily diet come from proteins.

You can also be very healthy as a vegetarian, eating occasional dairy, or even as a vegan, eating only plant-based foods. Plants contain all of the essential protein building blocks that you need. Vegetarians have a lower risk of cancer, heart disease, diabetes, obesity, and stroke. A review of 40 studies concluded that vegetarians also tend to weigh about 20 percent less than meat-eaters. If you're taking a prenatal vitamin (see page 81), you'll get an added boost in B vitamins that some vegetarians may need.

PRINCIPLE SEVEN:
MICRONUTRIENTS—FERTILITY-BOOSTING SUPPLEMENTS

Over the last 50 years, there has been a steady decline in the vitamin and mineral content of our foods, largely because of efforts to increase crop yields and speed the time to harvest—this doesn't give plants enough time to acquire adequate minerals from the soil, or produce as many nutrients. These efforts are less likely to occur on organic farms. By switching to an organically based diet, you'll be enhancing your nutrient and antioxidant intake. But you can also take certain supplements to improve your fertility and the health of your pregnancy. Each of the recommendations that follow is based on the latest scientific evidence. I recommend that women who are trying to get pregnant take a prenatal vitamin. But since they all don't contain adequate levels of the key nutrients I list below, be sure to supplement as needed.

One caveat: The supplement industry is currently an unregulated market, and some less-scrupulous companies may not produce supplements based on any standardization—some may contain less of a nutrient than the bottle claims, and some may be tainted. For instance, an alarming number of over-the-counter supplements have been found to contain lead. To protect yourself, only purchase products that say they pass testing by an independent agency like the United States Pharmacopeia (USP), National Sanitation Foundation (NSF), an international quality assurance testing agency, or ConsumerLab.

You and your partner would both benefit from increasing the following micronutrients through diet or taking a supplement. If you are taking a prenatal vitamin, check to make sure you're not duplicating any nutrients.

Vitamin C. Aside from its well-known cold-prevention benefits, vitamin C is involved in many bodily functions, including the breakdown of fats to release their calories. This helps you lose weight and keep you energized. Nearly 40 percent of adults in the United States have inadequate levels of vitamin C. By taking a supplement of 250 milligrams (mg) twice a day with meals, you'll release calories from fat about 45 percent more efficiently than if you weren't taking a supplement.

Vitamin D. This vitamin is often referred to as the "sunshine hormone," because we produce it in our skin when exposed to sunlight. If you always wear sunscreen, though, or if you have a dark complexion, you may not be producing enough. Vitamin D is vital to cells that use calcium, such as your intestines, bone-building cells, muscles, nerves, and immune system. Recently, low vitamin D levels have been linked to diabetes, as well as breast, colon, and prostate cancers. A review of 63 studies suggests that you should consume about 1,000 international units (IU) of vitamin D each day to prevent fatigue and bone loss—preferably in the form of vitamin D$_3$, or cholecalciferol.

Vitamin E. This potent antioxidant captures free radicals, protecting your cells from damage, including damage to DNA (see "Fertility Fact: Free Radicals Affect Fertility," page 66). Sperm are very susceptible to free radical damage. For women, about 20 to 30 IU per day should provide adequate protection, whereas men ought to aim for about 200 IU per day.

Calcium. About 99 percent of your calcium is stored in your teeth and bones. The remaining 1 percent circulates in your body and plays a critical role in promoting nerve signaling, muscle contractions, and hormone release—including insulin. If you take a calcium supplement with your meals, you'll reduce the absorption of fats in your food. This can help prevent the gain of about a pound per year, a benefit that can add up over time. Take 1,000 mg per day.

Magnesium. When magnesium is low, nerves become overly active and trigger the release of fight-or-flight hormones. This can set off a chain reaction that contributes to insulin resistance, depression, and compromised immune function. By getting about 400 mg per day, you'll lower your risk of diabetes by about 40 percent. If you eat a variety of fruits and vegetables, especially dark-green leafy vegetables, whole grains, bran, tofu, lentils, cashews, and wheat germ, then you don't need a supplement. If you don't regularly eat these foods, consider a supplement.

Iodine. This mineral is a vital component of your thyroid hormones. Because your body can't store iodine, you need to consume it on a daily basis, which is why it's added to table salt. Yet, according to the CDC, about 12 percent of Americans don't consume enough *iodide,* the dietary form of iodine, to support adequate thyroid hormone production. Iodine deficiency is the most common cause of low thyroid levels. Contributing to the problem is the growing popularity of gourmet salts like sea salt, most of which are not iodized. Always use iodized salt when cooking. You should try to get 150 micrograms (mcg) per day, the amount contained in about a half a teaspoon of iodized salt.

Chromium picolinate. This mineral improves insulin's ability to move glucose into targeted cells to be used as fuel, and it also reduces cravings. At doses of 200 mcg, three times each day, it has been shown to markedly reduce urges for comfort foods and increase the likelihood of ovulation in women with insulin resistance.

BEST ANTIOXIDANT FOOD SOURCES	
Fruits	◆ Blueberries ◆ Cranberries ◆ Pomegranate ◆ Blackberries ◆ Plums ◆ Dried plums ◆ Raspberries ◆ Strawberries ◆ Apples ◆ Citrus fruit
Vegetables	◆ Artichoke hearts ◆ Russet potatoes ◆ Spinach ◆ Sweet potatoes ◆ Tomatoes ◆ Bell peppers ◆ Winter squash ◆ Dark greens
Legumes	◆ Small red beans ◆ Red kidney beans ◆ Pinto beans ◆ Black beans
Nuts	◆ Pecans ◆ Walnuts ◆ Hazelnuts
Beverages	◆ Coffee ◆ Cocoa ◆ Tea (black and green)
Treats	◆ Dark chocolate

SUPPLEMENTS FOR HER

Prenatal vitamin. Begin taking your prenatal vitamin about three months before you start trying to conceive. A prenatal vitamin may not increase your chance of becoming pregnant, but it can improve the health of your pregnancy. One study showed that women who started a prenatal vitamin before they conceived had nearly a 75 percent reduction in the risk of developing *preeclampsia,* a potentially life-threatening complication of pregnancy. Your prenatal vitamin should contain at least 1 mg of folic acid to reduce the risk of birth defects like spina bifida and cleft palate in your child. It should also contain the B vitamins. Since not all prenatal vitamins contain the same combination of nutrients, I recommend the prescriptions Natelle Prefer, PrimaCare, Duet, OptiNate, or Citracal Prenatal 90+ DHA. PreCare Premier is a great choice for vegetarians because it has a higher dose of B vitamins than others. These prenatal vitamins may only be covered by insurance if you're pregnant. Avoid over-the-counter prenatal vitamins because they are not regulated by the FDA.

our story

Dr. Greene: After our IVF treatment failed, we decided to take a step back. Rather than try IVF again or even add on other high-tech procedures, we retreated to using ovulation-enhancement drugs along with intrauterine insemination—this is considered a basic fertility treatment rather than an advanced treatment. But before even trying another cycle of this, we wanted to optimize everything we could about our diet to improve our hormone balance even more. We are both vegetarians, so we already followed the Perfect Balance plan, but there's always room for improvement. Morgan made an extra effort to avoid unhealthy fats and processed foods, and we cut back on going out for dinner. Morgan also started taking DHA, an omega-3 supplement, and I began taking ConceptionXR, the male fertility supplement. After waiting six months, we did two cycles of the basic treatment and Morgan became pregnant on the second try. I have no doubt that these minor changes contributed to our success.

Omega-3 fatty acid supplements. These contain essential fatty acids, oils that you need to maintain healthy nerves and a healthy immune system. Your body can't manufacture these, so if you're not getting enough through diet, you're at a higher risk for depression, heart disease, rheumatoid arthritis, and diabetes. They're even more important to the development of your baby once you become pregnant. It's absolutely essential that you get omega-3 into your diet. Unfortunately, the richest source of these healthy oils is fish, but fish contain so many toxins that can harm a fetus—such as mercury, lead, and dioxins—that you should avoid them while you're trying to conceive and while you're pregnant. I recommend that you consider eating about a tablespoon of ground flaxseed each day, which you can sprinkle on your cereal or salad. If you don't like the taste of flax, try Smart Balance butter substitute or peanut butter, eggs fortified with DHA, and walnuts. Or consider a supplement made from algae like Expecta LIPIL.

SUPPLEMENTS FOR HIM

The simplest option for men is to take ConceptionXR, a supplement that contains appropriate amounts of the following nutrients plus some of the other nutrients listed in the recommendations for both of you.

Folic acid. Testicles use folic acid to make DNA for their prolific production of sperm. Studies show that even fertile men can have improved sperm production by taking a supplement of 5 mg of folic acid each day along with a zinc supplement (see below).

Zinc. Trace amounts of zinc improve sperm formation, testosterone metabolism, and sperm motility. According to studies, taking 10 mg per day can boost sperm production and improve pregnancy rates.

Selenium. This mineral acts as an antioxidant, and helps insulin to move glucose out of the bloodstream and cells. It has also been shown to increase sperm motility. Try to get about 200 mcg per day,

A FEW MORE SUPPLEMENTS TO CONSIDER

The following supplements have also been well researched and shown to improve sperm function. There isn't evidence that everyone needs these like they do the micronutrients, but if you suspect that you have a male fertility problem, you may be able to enhance your sperm function by taking one. Once you go on to consider treatment, discuss with your fertility specialist whether you should continue any of these. As with other supplement recommendations, look for the USP or NSF label to be sure of the purity and dose-to-dose consistency of anything you purchase.

◆ **Flaxseed (linseed) oil** contains two important ingredients: *alpha-linolenic acid (ALA)* and *lignans.* Studies show that men with infertility tend to have lower ALA in their daily diet. This dietary oil increases the fluidity of the sperm membrane and its ability to interact with the oocyte. During digestion, lignans generate metabolites that reduce the conversion of testosterone to estradiol, shifting a man's hormone balance in a more fertile direction. Dosage studies are not clear, so consider a 1,000 mg capsule daily—the standard dose.

◆ **Astacarox** is made from the alga *Haematococcus pluvialis* and has a strong antioxidant effect. Studies have shown that 16 mg per day reduced free radical formation in the semen and lowered the production of the hormone inhibin-B, a natural inhibiter of sperm production. The key ingredient is believed to be a chemical called astaxanthin.

◆ **Pycnogenol** is an herbal supplement extracted from the bark of the *Pinus maritima* tree. Studies found that 200 mg taken once a day can double the percentage of normal sperm produced in men with low sperm counts. It is believed to work as both an antioxidant and an anti-inflammatory.

either from a supplement or by eating three to four Brazil nuts twice a week. Brown rice, walnuts, and whole wheat bread are also good sources of selenium.

Lycopene. This powerful antioxidant and natural pigment is abundant in tomatoes. Recent studies have found high levels of lycopene in healthy male testicles, suggesting a protective effect. Low levels are associated with infertility and a higher risk of prostate cancer. If you don't eat about a small raw tomato or about half a cup of tomato sauce every day, consider a supplement with about 5 mg of lycopene each day to help protect your sperm from free radical damage.

Carnitine (or L-carnitine). This micronutrient, made from the amino acid lysine, is produced in the liver, the brain, and the kidneys. It shuttles fatty acids into the part of the cell where they are broken down to release energy. Since the testicles don't make adequate amounts of carnitine to meet the needs of sperm, they rely on what's released by the liver. Carnitine has been shown to be most useful in men with a low sperm count. I recommend 500 mg twice each day and would consider increasing the dose to three times a day if there is no improvement after three months.

◆　◆　◆

As you make these changes to your diet, you'll begin to feel more energetic and have a greater sense of well-being. People say they can really feel the difference when their blood sugar, for instance, isn't jumping up and down. Hunger is more manageable and your energy level will be more consistent. Your body will take notice as well. In some people, these dietary changes can help balance their hormones to the point that they can get pregnant without any treatment. But don't stop here. The exercise and stress-reducing advice I offer in the next two chapters also play important roles in hormone balance and your fertility.

5 Shaping Up to Promote Pregnancy

I'd like you to begin to think of exercise not as having "benefits" for your health and fertility, but as being a necessity. Your level of exercise, and your partner's, may be directly related to your level of fertility, especially for those who are at the activity extremes—the sedentary and the ultra-active. Throughout history, our ability to survive and reproduce has been closely linked to our ability to move—our ability to gather, hunt, and produce food, to journey to more plentiful lands, and to evade predators. Our bodies have many built-in mechanisms that help us to adapt to physical demands, and most of these adaptations are driven by hormones. For instance, when we become active, the antidiuretic hormone is released to help prevent dehydration, fight-or-flight hormones rise to shift our blood flow to our muscles, and a variety of rest-and-digest hormones dip as we switch into calorie-burning mode. But as good as we are at adjusting to physical challenges, our bodies adapt poorly to a lack of activity. Survival was never based on our being still. Just look at the results of the inactivity that pervades our society today. As we have led more mechanized and sedentary lives, we've experienced a steady rise in obesity, diabetes, and heart disease—and infertility.

At the other extreme, being overactive can affect your fertility as well. With the popularity of marathons and various extreme sports, many very fit women may find that their menstrual cycles either stop or

Case in Point

I hadn't seen Jeff in nearly six years. At that time, his wife, Gina, had come to me to reverse her tubal ligation so they could have their first child together. She had her "tubes tied" in her previous marriage. When their child was about five, they tried to become pregnant again, but after a year, they came back to my office. When they walked in, I was surprised at how much weight Jeff had gained. He explained that he had suffered a back injury from a car accident and became sedentary. Since his injury, Jeff had gained nearly 70 pounds. I did a workup of Gina, who was 36, and found no problems with her fertility.

I explained that Jeff had to resume regular exercise and restore a healthy diet. I also recommended that he take the multivitamin ConceptionXR to support his sperm production. I referred Jeff to a physical therapist so he could learn ways of exercising that wouldn't worsen his back problem, and recommended a balanced program of aerobic exercise, strength training, and gentle yoga. Jeff had also been taking frequent saunas to relieve his back pain, but this was exposing his testicles to high heat and likely reducing sperm production. I suggested he use localized heat therapy on his back instead.

When they returned for their three-month follow-up, the difference was remarkable. Jeff had lost 28 pounds and his sperm count improved considerably. Jeff also confided that his libido had returned. Two months later, Gina was pregnant again. She delivered a healthy baby girl.

become irregular. Men may experience a decline in sperm count. This reflects a shift in your hormones that redirects calories toward supporting your extreme physical feats rather than promoting reproduction.

WHY MOVING MATTERS

Preventing insulin resistance is a key benefit of exercise, though there are many other subtle benefits that I will come back to in a moment. Recall that muscles take in glucose from the bloodstream with the help of insulin. Muscles store glucose as glycogen—the short-term energy that they use on an as-needed basis. Exercise not only builds muscles, but makes them more efficient at taking in glucose, so less insulin is

HOW VALUABLE IS EXERCISE?

Studies have shown that 30 minutes of daily aerobic exercise can lower a number of health risks:

1. Breast cancer is reduced by 20 to 30 percent.
2. Colon cancer is reduced by 30 to 50 percent.
3. Type 2 diabetes is reduced by 30 to 40 percent.
4. Osteoporosis is reduced by 50 percent.
5. Stroke is reduced by 30 to 50 percent.
6. Heart disease is reduced by 40 to 50 percent.
7. Premature death is reduced by 30 to 50 percent.

needed to help keep blood sugar levels stable. With low insulin levels, you have a reduced risk of insulin resistance. Studies show that about 45 minutes of exercise will reduce insulin resistance for about 36 hours. Also, muscles that have been exercised remain packed with glycogen, providing them with lots of strength and vigor.

Sedentary people, by contrast, have smaller, inefficient muscles, and therefore rely more heavily on insulin to help pump glucose into the muscles, setting the stage for insulin resistance.

But this isn't the only benefit of exercising.

Exercise lowers stress hormones (known impediments to fertility), improves blood flow to the pelvic area so that the uterus and ovaries have plenty of oxygen, improves immune function by lowering inflammation (which can interfere with implantation), helps fight fatigue so you have more energy to be sexually responsive, and normalizes your circadian rhythm (your body's internal clock) so that you sleep more soundly. Deep sleep promotes nighttime hormone production and ovulation, and helps lower stress. As your fitness improves, you'll find that you are in a better mood, have more energy, have fewer aches, and enjoy a more fulfilling sex life—all ingredients to a more fertile you.

Did you know ?

Exercise promotes antioxidants that help limit the damage that free radicals can inflict on the DNA of eggs and sperm.

THE HORMONE PLAYERS

Just as food choices impact your hormones, so does your activity level. The difference is that your diet mainly impacts hormones that store energy, whereas exercise releases hormones that *burn* energy.

♦ **Glucagon** signals the liver to release glucose whenever blood sugar drops, particularly during exercise.

♦ **Growth hormone (GH),** like glucagon, frees glucose from the liver, and also promotes the growth of cartilage, bones, and muscles, and encourages fat to be used as fuel. The biggest surge in GH comes from moderate exercise—the intensity that boosts your heart rate and challenges your endurance.

♦ **Insulin-like growth factor (IGF-1)** works with GH to keep sugar from dipping too low. Exercise can naturally boost IGF-1.

♦ **Testosterone.** Exercise increases testosterone levels, which boost glycogen storage in muscles, muscle strength, endurance, and libido.

♦ **Estrogen.** Exercising helps balance estrogen levels. Women who are overweight, sedentary, or in their later reproductive years tend to have higher-than-normal levels of estrone, a "bad" estrogen, creating an imbalance that may suppress estradiol's signal to ovulate (estrone competes with estradiol for receptors, weakening estradiol's effect). Exercise helps shed fat, and because fat cells produce estrone, having smaller fat cells means there's less estrone to interfere with estradiol's functions. Overexercising, though, can lower estradiol levels, too, and result in a reduced chance of implantation.

PERFECT BALANCE EXERCISE PLAN

In the last chapter, you determined how many calories you needed to increase or cut back on in order to gain or lose weight. If you increase the intensity or length of time you exercise, you'll burn more calories each day. Weight management is a matter of balancing the calories you take in with the calories you expend. The following table lists the approximate number of calories burned for men and women during 30 minutes of a specific activity, based on your weight. Use this table as an estimate of calories burned, since actual calories burned can vary among individuals.

Before you get started, write down your fitness and weight goals in an exercise log. Document your weight, your resting heart rate (to deter-

CALORIES BURNED PER 30 MINUTES OF ACTIVITY BASED ON YOUR WEIGHT (LBS)

Activity	Weight				
	120	140	160	180	200
Aerobics (high-impact)	201	223	255	286	311
Aerobics (low-impact)	158	181	198	233	252
Circuit training (with weights)	230	249	268	293	327
Cycling (12 mph)	230	249	268	293	327
Elliptical trainer	259	281	303	324	346
Gardening	130	141	152	163	174
Kayaking	144	156	171	189	207
Rowing machine	210	226	244	263	282
Running (10-minute-mile pace)	173	188	204	221	243
Sex (average exertion)	105	134	154	172	193
Stair climber	173	173	188	204	221
Swimming (freestyle)	173	188	204	221	243
Walking (flat, 17-minute-mile pace)	115	125	138	147	159
Water aerobics	115	125	138	147	159
Weight training	97	115	124	135	146
Yoga, hatha	115	125	138	147	159

Ask Dr. Greene

Q Can my menstrual cycles affect my athletic performance?

A Yes. Depending on what sport you're playing, your menstrual cycles can impact your performance. Several studies have demonstrated that monthly hormonal fluctuations have minimal impact on strength specific sports like weight lifting or intense anaerobic ones like sprint racing. However, other studies show that your performance in endurance sports can definitely be compromised during the last two weeks of your cycle. These effects are exacerbated in hot weather. Keep in mind, too, that endurance sports can have the most negative impact on your chance of becoming pregnant when taken to the extremes.

mine this, see page 39), and how much you currently exercise, as well as where you'd like to be in three months. Then repeat these measurements every month to track your progress.

PRINCIPLE ONE: START A BALANCED EXERCISE PROGRAM

Every program should incorporate aerobic activity, strength-building exercises, and flexibility training. Try to alternate among a variety of activities that you enjoy to stay motivated and prevent exercise burnout. If you are currently inactive, it typically takes two to three months to achieve a healthy level of fitness. Be sure to consult with your physician if you're starting an exercise program for the first time.

If you need help getting started, ask for a referral to a physical therapist or a qualified personal trainer.

1. **Aerobic activity.** Healthy functioning of your heart, cardiovascular system, and lungs is built on activities that require a constant oxygen supply—the defining characteristic of aerobic exercise. Your ideal goal is to perform aerobic activity for 40 to 60 minutes per day. If you are new to aerobic exercise, start with 20 minutes a day and gradually increase to 30, or you can break it up into two to three 20-minute sessions.

Types of aerobic activity include:
- Walking
- Jogging
- Running
- Cycling

- Kickboxing
- Stair climbing
- Step classes
- Swimming
- Dancing

2. **Strength training.** This builds muscles and strengthens bones. Bigger muscles help burn calories, even when you're not exercising, because it takes more energy to sustain muscle cells than it does fat cells. Choose one or two exercises that target each of the large muscle groups— chest, shoulders, back, arms, abdomen, quadriceps, hamstrings, gluteus (buttocks), and calves. Build your training program slowly to prevent injury. Work toward doing 8 to 12 repetitions of 8 to 10 exercises per session. To maintain your muscle strength, do strength training twice a week, allowing two days of rest in between workouts. To build muscle, aim for three days a week.

Types of strength-training exercises include:
- Free weights (dumbbells)
- Gym machines (Nautilus)
- Resistance bands
- Fitness balls
- Isometric (pushing against a stationery object)
- Strength training group classes
- Power yoga
- Push-ups, sit-ups, and pull-ups
- Climbing

Ask Dr. Greene

Q Can I continue exercising once I'm pregnant?

A Your doctor should insist upon it. Over the last 15 years, there has been a paradigm shift in thinking. Women have traditionally been discouraged from exercising during their pregnancy. Research has revealed, though, that being sedentary during pregnancy promotes excessive weight gain, blood pressure problems, and gestational diabetes. It also contributes to lifelong problems for your developing child, such as a higher risk of childhood obesity. That's why the American College of Obstetricians and Gynecologists currently recommends at least 45 to 60 minutes of exercise every day of pregnancy.

3. **Flexibility and balance.** This is the most overlooked of all fitness categories. Stretching improves the range of motion of your joints and muscles to improve coordination, reduce the incidence of injury, and help maintain agility. Incorporate flexibility training into your fitness program three days a week for 20 to 30 minutes and do a five-minute stretch after exercising.

Did you know ?

Drinking a sports drink high in carbs while exercising reduces the number of fat calories you burn since your body simply uses the calories from the beverage for energy. Hydrate with water or other noncaloric drinks instead.

Activities that promote balance and flexibility include:

◆ Yoga
◆ Tai chi
◆ Surfing or skateboarding
◆ Pilates

You can also choose an activity that combines flexibility with strength or endurance. These "hybrids" include:

◆ Power yoga (yoga + strength training)
◆ Tae bo (tai chi + aerobic kickboxing)
◆ Cyclates (spinning + Pilates)

PRINCIPLE TWO: ACTIVATE YOUR LIFESTYLE

Being active during your "downtime" is equally important as the time you spend working out at the gym or outdoors. Just how significant this downtime is came to light in a study that looked at why some people were more resistant to weight gain than others when placed on high-calorie diets. When researchers gave a group of students an extra 1,000 calories per day for a month, the students that were very active when doing "nothing" did not gain weight. The calories they burned informally by standing, fidgeting, walking, or maintaining good posture were enough to offset the extra caloric load. In fact, they burned the equivalent of several hours of walking each day. Another study found that obese people spent about two hours more each day sitting than those who maintained a healthy weight.

By activating your lifestyle, you can burn an extra 350 calories per day. Here are a few suggestions for starters; use them to fuel your own ideas.

EXERCISE: A POTENT ANTI-INFLAMMATORY

Whenever you're injured or sick, various cells in your body produce inflammatory chemicals that activate your immune system. This reaction can actually block the release of a mature egg by your ovaries and prevent the implantation of a fertilized egg in your womb. Exercise temporarily increases inflammation, but when performed on a regular basis, it has the opposite effect. Regular daily exercise enhances your immune system so it can repair injuries without the systemic release of these inflammatory chemicals. Add this to the list of fertility-boosting effects of exercise.

- *Spend less time sitting.* Get a headset so you can get up and pace in your office when you're talking on the phone.
- *Increase your walking pace when running errands.*
- *Park a little farther away.* Instead of circling the parking lot looking for that ideal spot by the door, take the one at the end of the lot to give you a chance to stretch your legs.
- *Fidget* when you're stuck in traffic or at your desk. If you don't typically fidget, it entails tapping a foot, drumming your fingers, twirling your hair, and other mindless movements.
- *Chew sugarless gum* to burn about 11 calories per hour. As an added bonus, gum chewing boosts blood flow to your brain, which can make you feel more alert.
- *Sign up for dance lessons.* Trade an evening of watching TV for dance lessons with your partner. It might be a welcome diversion from your daily routine and will improve muscle strength, balance, and coordination.
- *Take the stairs.* You can burn from 5 to 10 calories per flight of stairs. Even if you take one or two flights twice a day, the benefits will add up.
- *Sit up straight.* We tend to have lazy habits with our posture. Sitting up straight requires your core muscles to work and burn more calories.
- *Take an evening walk.* The fastest way to trigger hormonal imbalance is to go directly from the dinner table to the couch. If you take an evening walk instead, you'll store your calories in your muscles, not your fat cells.

CYCLING: A POTENTIAL FERTILITY RISK

If cycling is your sport, the bicycle seat may pose a risk to your fertility. The pudendal nerves and arteries that support sexual function pass between the skin and bony surface of your "sit bones" (ischial and pubic bones). As a result, the time spent on a hard narrow seat, compounded by the jostling impact, creates a risk of sexual dysfunction as well as difficulty urinating. Because men have a narrower pelvis, their risk is greater. To reduce risk while trying to conceive, take the following steps.

◆ **Purchase an ergonomically shaped gel seat.** These are designed to reduce pressure on the sit bones. They are shaped differently for women and men, so consult a bike shop to find the best seat for you.

◆ **Shorten your rides** so you're not pushing the limits. If you're experiencing numbness, stop riding for the day.

◆ **Consider switching to mountain biking** since you'll spend more time standing on your pedals, less time in the saddle. Studies also show that the body position used in mountain biking relieves pressure on the nerves and blood vessels of the genitals.

◆ **Men should avoid tight-fitting Lycra bike shorts.** They can raise the temperature of the testicles and sperm, potentially leading to lower sperm count.

◆ **Consult a urologist or gynecologist** if you're already experiencing symptoms of numbness, sexual dysfunction, or difficulty urinating. Saddle-related problems tend to resolve within three to six months.

PRINCIPLE THREE: CUT BACK IF YOU EXERCISE TOO MUCH

While trying to get pregnant, it's much easier to cross the line from healthy exercising to overexercising. Pushing your body too hard, too long, or too often can reduce your chances of conception. Overtraining, for most people, is defined as the level and intensity of exercise that exceeds your body's ability to recover. Warning signs can include prolonged fatigue after your workout, chronic mild muscle soreness, sleep disturbances, elevated resting heart rate, missed menstrual cycles, and increased incidence of injuries. The very fit may not experience these symptoms, but may be compromising their fertility nonetheless.

One recent study found that fit adults who had infertility and were participating in vigorous exercise like running for at least four hours each week had a marked reduction in their success when going through IVF. In fact, the women that had been working out for more than nine years at this level had the lowest success rate in the study. These findings suggest that for people who are normal weight and very fit, it's very easy to tip the balancing benefits of exercise too far and create problems. Keep in mind that these results only reflect women with infertility who were normal weight. But the broader message is that moderation is key when it comes to vigorous exercise. If you think you may be overdoing it, or if you have any of the warning signs mentioned above, begin to cut back. Take a moment to jot down your symptoms in your exercise log, and document your daily efforts to cut back (be sure not to relax so much that you're not exercising at all). Here are some great ways to cut back without losing your fitness benefits.

- Limit *vigorous* exercise such as running, aerobics class, or any high-intensity activity to no more than three one-hour sessions a week.
- If you want more workout time, replace some of your vigorous activities with strength training and less-intense exercises, like yoga, which have not been shown to trigger the hormonal imbalances that may contribute to infertility.
- Focus on form and improving your skill level rather than speed or endurance.
- Take a break. Give your muscles and joints a few days to rest and regenerate.
- If exercise is the only way you deal with stress, find other coping mechanisms to turn to some of the time (see chapter 6).

PRINCIPLE FOUR: CREATE LONG-TERM CHANGE

The most important goal of your fitness program is to make exercise a habit rather than a short-term effort. The best way to achieve this is to seek out activities that you enjoy. Today, there is an ever-increasing number of sports and exercise classes to participate in. Try a new activity for inspiration. Brain researchers have found that the brain's pleasure center lights up when someone engages in something new. Here are some other tips to help you stay motivated.

- *Listen to music during your workouts.* Music can trigger your brain's emotional center. Choose songs with a fast beat—you'll pick up the pace and find that the time passes more quickly.

- *Create a healthy addiction.* Work out to the point of breathlessness for at least 20 minutes during aerobic activities—at this level, your brain releases endorphins, responsible for the "runner's high."
- *Stay hydrated.* Drink enough fluid to replace what you lose through your perspiration to keep your energy level high. If you wait until you feel thirsty, you'll already be dehydrated and approaching fatigue.
- *Consider a personal trainer.* If you need some guidance, hire a fitness pro to get off to a strong start. There are several organizations that certify fitness instructors, like the Aerobics and Fitness Association of America, so check out a trainer's credentials before you make a commitment.
- *Check your fitness diary to track your progress.* When you reach a goal, reward yourself—with a massage rather than an ice cream!
- *Find a fitness buddy.* It's much harder to talk yourself out of a workout when someone else is depending on you. Seek out someone with similar fitness goals and interests so that you provide each other with support rather than competition. Even better, try to find someone dealing with fertility issues. You'll both benefit from the emotional support, and may learn from each other's fertility experiences. Contact national organizations such as RESOLVE (www.resolve.org) or the American Fertility Association (www.theafa.org), or contact a local support group for infertility.

◆　◆　◆

Your energy level is going to improve as you modify your fitness routine. As you become more (or less) active, track changes in your menstrual cycle and libido. You'll likely notice the symptoms of hormonal imbalance slowly fading, which can be a big psychological boost in your efforts to get pregnant. The third component of your Perfect Balance program is dealing with stress. In the next chapter, I offer a variety of effective stress management tools to help reduce your stress hormone level.

6 Coping with Stress to Boost Fertility

Chances are a friend has told you the anecdote of the couple who tried multiple fertility treatments without success, finally decided to adopt, and the next thing they knew they became pregnant. The well-meaning but misguided message: Once you stop stressing about trying to get pregnant, you will conceive. The problem with this fairy-tale ending is that it just doesn't happen to everyone who goes on to adopt. There is, however, truth to the stress-fertility connection. The research clearly shows that stress contributes to infertility. Chronic stress can cause menstrual irregularity, which can interfere with ovulation, and it can create subtler hormonal changes that interfere with reproduction in other ways. Yet, there are few things more stressful to most couples than dealing with fertility troubles, potentially causing a snowball effect. Men are also susceptible to the fertility-robbing effects of stress, though less so than women. Large studies of infertility patients have found that male stress reduces success rates, and studies of men who participated in high-stress military training found suppressed

Did you know ?

Stress can have a cumulative effect on you as a couple—studies found that self-described high-stress couples have a two to three times greater rate of miscarriage.

Case in Point

A year after the birth of her first child, Liz was diagnosed with premature menopause at the age of 30. Since her mother experienced menopause at 35, Liz figured this was part of her family history and her destiny. She and her husband, Jon, went to a reproductive endocrinologist to see if there was any way that she could produce mature eggs to have a second child, but the doctor told her their only option was to use an egg donor. They decided not to pursue this, and accepted their family as it was.

Not long after this decision, Liz came to my office to talk about relieving her menopausal symptoms. She was surprised when I told her I questioned her diagnosis and that her blood tests were inconclusive. I explained that although she did have secondary amenorrhea—a loss of menstrual cycles—I wasn't convinced that she was menopausal. During her consultation, Liz told me about the work-related stress she was under. We discussed some of the relaxation methods she could use to reduce the stress in her life, such as yoga and meditation. I also encouraged her to follow my Perfect Balance program to try to get back to her prepregnancy weight (she had gained 60 pounds after her first pregnancy). Finally, I recommended she use a birth control pill, Yasmin, for six months, as an oral contraceptive can sometimes re-create the natural monthly cycle and improve the development of maturing eggs.

Liz was incredulous when she called me nine months later to share the news that she was pregnant. After stopping the birth control pills, her cycles had become regular. She had lost 35 pounds, had been practicing yoga regularly, and was handling her work stress more effectively. Because of her newfound health and well-being, she had stopped worrying about getting pregnant, and was just focusing on being healthy and feeling great. She gave birth to a healthy son.

testosterone levels for weeks after completing training exercises. Stress is also a major contributor to loss of libido and erectile dysfunction.

I know that telling couples simply to relax and not worry so much can only cause more frustration and anxiety. Telling them to eliminate stressors may be empty words—most people don't have the luxury of leaving a stressful job, for instance. The focus of this chapter is to give you evidence-based tools that have been shown to lower stress hormone levels, and to provide you with recommendations for reducing your personal reaction to stressors. By getting your stress under control now, you may be able to avoid fertility treatment. But if that alone is insufficient, the coping skills you'll learn will help keep stress at bay as you go through treatments, if you choose to do so.

YOUR BODY'S RESPONSE TO STRESS

Our perception of what is stressful differs from one person to the next, and we all have different ways of coping with stressors. In these ways, our stress response is highly individualized. But when we do perceive a threatening situation, our bodies all respond with a predictable series of hormone-brain interactions.

Typically, a number of events happen almost simultaneously when you're under stress, but there are three main hormone-brain connections at play.

> **Did you know ?**
>
> Current brain imaging research suggests that our sensitivity to stress is related to how our brain produces the feel-good neurotransmitter serotonin. People with less serotonin are more sensitive to stressors.

1. **The sympathetic nervous system.** Your brain sends messages via the sympathetic nervous system, a special set of nerves that have the sole function of setting off an alarm. This system provides direct communication from the brain to other parts of your body and is faster acting than the hormone message system described above. These nerves go to fat cells, where they trigger the release of calories, to the heart, where they instantly increase your heart rate, and to the skin, where they can trigger nervous sweating. Most important, nerves that go to the adrenal gland stimulate the release of adrenaline.

2. **The hypothalamic-pituitary-adrenal axis** is the hormone brain circuit that initiates the stress response. The brain's hypothalamus triggers the pituitary gland, the brain's hormone shipping department, to release a hormone called *corticotrophin-releasing hormone (CRH)* that travels to the adrenal glands, where it triggers the release of cortisol.

3. **The pain relief system.** Simultaneously, the hypothalamus also promotes the release of pain-relieving endorphins that course through your body.

THE HORMONE PLAYERS

The stress response is an adaptive, helpful response to a perceived threat. It only becomes harmful if your stress is chronic. Here are the key hormones that are released during stress, along with their immediate benefits and long-term hazards.

Hormone	Immediate Benefits	Long-term Hazards
Epinephrine (adrenaline)	It's mainly responsible for the fight-or-flight response—that shot of stimulation that courses through your body when you narrowly avoid a car accident. It boosts heart rate, raises blood sugar, turns down the immune response, and shifts blood away from your skin, digestive system, and reproductive organs and toward large muscles to promote strength. It only circulates briefly in response to a danger.	It can contribute to high blood pressure and generalized anxiety.
Cortisol	Like adrenaline, it causes a rise in blood pressure, raises blood sugar, and shuts down the immune system in response to a perceived danger. Cortisol can remain elevated for weeks or months. Cortisol levels are naturally lowest in the early evening and highest shortly before waking each morning.	It can suppress your immune system, raise blood sugar and blood pressure, and reduce fertility by inhibiting the maturation of eggs and sperm. It can also contribute to depression.
Endorphins	These are your body's natural pain relievers that are released under stress.	They become less effective at pain relief, and can inhibit the production of sperm and the maturation of eggs.
Prolactin	It's best known for its role in releasing breast milk. Experts don't know why it's also released under stress, but believe it is involved in bonding between people in a dangerous situation. It may also help ease some of the negative emotional effects of stress.	It may block ovulation and lower sperm production. Some studies suggest it contributes to infertility in about one-third of couples with "unexplained fertility." When chronically elevated, it may interfere with bonding.

TIME TO RECONSIDER THAT NIPPLE PIERCING OR BREAST SURGERY

An often overlooked trigger for prolactin release is nipple and breast stimulation. As more women and men choose to wear body jewelry, we are learning more about their effects. Immediately after a nipple piercing and sometimes for months afterward, a man's sperm count and libido may drop, whereas women may develop irregular menstrual cycles or anovulatory ones (you get your period but don't ovulate). Similarly, the recovery phase from any breast surgery can also prompt a temporary or prolonged interruption in fertility. If you've already had a procedure, consider having your prolactin level tested, but request the test first thing in the morning, on an empty stomach, to measure your baseline level.

Because of the many complex systems involved, the stress response has been difficult to study. Some people respond to stress by activating each of these systems, whereas others may only activate one stress response. It has also been shown that people that are under chronic stress tend to have a more exaggerated response when a new danger or obstacle is encountered. Those that have more effective coping mechanisms are able to diminish the stress response quicker and prevent chronic stress from contributing to health problems.

COMMON TYPES OF STRESS

We tend to think of stress as emotional, but physiological and environmental factors can also stress our bodies.

Physiological	Emotional	Environmental
Inadequate calories	Relationship issues	Pesticides/herbicides
Prolonged cold temperature	Financial pressures	Pollution
Excessive heat	Work-related stress	Secondhand smoke
Exercise to exhaustion	Infertility	Processed foods
Insufficient sleep	Sexual dysfunction	Impure water
Infection	Feeling helpless	Occupational hazards
Injury/trauma	Family health	Computer terminals

PERFECT BALANCE MIND-BODY PLAN

There are many ways to reduce and cope with stress, but before you read on, take the Perfect Balance Stress Test below to assess how it's affecting you on a day-to-day basis, and how much you need to focus on reducing stress in your life. Re-take the test once a month if you feel your stress level rising.

Of all the stress-reducing methods, the following are the best researched and most effective in improving hormone balance, which can set the stage for conception. Not every method fits every personal-

PERFECT BALANCE STRESS TEST					
	Always (4)	Often (3)	Regularly (2)	Sometimes (1)	Never (0)
Do you have indigestion?	4	3	2	1	0
Do you feel lonely?	4	3	2	1	0
Are you unusually susceptible to illnesses?	4	3	2	1	0
Do you feel anxious?	4	3	2	1	0
Have your sleep patterns changed— do you sleep too much or too little?	4	3	2	1	0
Do you feel betrayed?	4	3	2	1	0
Do you worry a lot compared to your friends or family?	4	3	2	1	0
Do you feel shy or timid?	4	3	2	1	0
Do you seek out friendships and social situations?	4	3	2	1	0

Total your score. Here's the bottom line:

10 or less: Your stress levels are pretty low. You're coping well!

11–20: Not bad, but you might improve your fertility if you practiced one or more of the upcoming mind-balancing techniques.

21–30: Your stress hormones are getting the better of you. You need to take time out of your schedule to relax and get back on an even keel to improve your reproductive health.

31–40: Call to action! Your stress hormones could be seriously interfering with your fertility. Make your emotional health a priority. Promise yourself to take time out of every day for relaxation.

ity, so try the ones that appeal to you. Come back to this chapter if you ultimately need fertility treatment to consider additional ways you can better quiet your worries and trigger your relaxation response during treatment.

PRINCIPLE ONE: CHOOSE A RELAXATION EXERCISE

We've all experienced that "muscle-tensing" sensation of stress, but when chronic stress occurs, the ongoing muscle tension can send the brain misleading information that the threat is still present, even though it has passed. The best way to correct this miscommunica-

tion is through meditation. There are many forms of meditation, but their goals are similar—to focus your mind on internal sensations and actions like breathing, while keeping out thoughts that are distracting. Brain imaging studies show that regions of the brain linked to happiness, empathy, and maternal bonding have increased activity even in novices beginning meditation training. With practice, these changes in personality traits become even more permanent.

The ancient practice of meditation gained its first dose of respect in mainstream medicine in 1972, when it was found to reverse many of the effects of stress. Since then, brain imaging studies have revealed that during meditation, the brain "rewires" connections between nerves to overcome a variety of unhealthy conditions like depression, anxiety, and attention-deficit/hyperactivity disorder (ADHD).

Studies have also found that meditative practices can consistently trigger the *relaxation response*—effectively turning off the stress response. The relaxation response has been shown to reduce the heart rate, slow breathing, and slow metabolism—all triggered by a reduction in fight-or-flight hormones and an increase in rest-and-digest hormones. But I know from discussions with my patients that because we live in an action-oriented society, many of us have trouble with lengthy sessions of seated meditation. If you fall into this category, consider one

<table>
<tr><td>

our story

Morgan: I knew I was feeling stressed out at work, but I tend to internalize my emotions and did not even think about how the stress of infertility might be exacerbating my work-related stress. Robert is an avid yoga fan, and he gently, albeit repeatedly, suggested I try it to relieve my stress. I resisted for many months. Yoga felt like one more thing to add to an already busy schedule that I had no interest in expanding. But after our IVF cycle proved unsuccessful, I agreed to a "trial run." It took about a month before I reached the point where I felt like I no longer had to force myself out the door to get to yoga class. But after that time, I started to look forward to class and the opportunity to let go and unwind. The longer I stayed with it, the longer those positive feelings remained after class and into the following day. Five months later, I was pregnant, and I thought, at the very least, yoga helped relieve my stress, and perhaps it did help me get pregnant.

</td></tr>
</table>

of the following techniques that have demonstrated similar efficacy at lowering stress.

Yoga has become one of the most popular and healthiest trends in the United States. This exercise-meditative practice that originated in India centuries ago combines stretching exercises and deep breathing. There are numerous styles of yoga, but I recommend that you seek out hatha yoga, a relaxing form of synchronized movement and breathing that doesn't focus on meditation, yet achieves similar results. In fact, there are a growing number of hatha-based "yoga-for-fertility" classes that might also give you the opportunity to meet other couples facing the same challenge. Encourage your partner to join you, as he can benefit from the stress-reducing effects as well. Studies show that a 45-minute session twice a week can dramatically reduce the effects of stress and promote hormone balance.

Walking meditation is an easy form of contemplative exercise in which your movement becomes the focus of your thoughts. Rather than completely tuning out your environment, as you would do during seated meditation, you are tuning in to your own movement. As you focus in on your body, you'll find that you will clear your mind of other thoughts. Start with 20 minutes and follow these instructions:

RELIGION AND INFERTILITY

Infertility can have a powerful impact on a person's faith and spirituality. One study of people who identified themselves as religious found that 25 percent of couples became more religious while dealing with infertility, but about 10 percent became less so. When they probed further, the researchers found that when the tenets of the religion were not supportive of fertility treatments or being infertile, couples turned away from their religion. Some faiths accept treatment as part of the wonder of modern living, whereas others view infertility as a form of punishment.

I bring this controversial topic up because many of my patients have experienced a negative response from their religious community, and I'd like to help you avoid that experience. I've had patients tell me that their clergy's unsupportive response to their struggle felt like a "slap on the face." Before you consider speaking with a clergy member or otherwise opening up about your issues, it's important to explore the position of your faith so that you're not put off or surprised by the response. If your religion is supportive, however, turning toward your place of worship for support may boost your fertility. One study found that people with a greater sense of spiritual well-being conceived quicker and experienced fewer symptoms of depression than others.

* Begin by standing still. Experience the way the soles of your feet interact with the ground to distribute your weight. Think about the subtle movements required to maintain your balance and remain upright.
* Start walking at a slow but comfortable pace. Continue to focus your attention on the soles of your feet—feel the subtle changes that take place from one step to the next.
* Keep your ankles loose and think about how gravity moves your feet as they transition from one step to the next. Then shift your focus to your knees, and finally to your hips. Exaggerate the movements of various muscle groups to help you focus on their unique qualities.
* If your thoughts wander, start over by returning your attention back on the soles of your feet and working your way up.
* Coordinate your breath with your movements. Alternate between keeping your hands clasped behind your back and moving them in unison with your legs, noting how your body feels switching from one style of walking to the other—this keeps the mind focused.

- Complete your meditation with a few moments of concentrated standing again. Note the difference in how your muscles and joints feel at rest after exercise compared to before.
- Modify your walks in length, time of day, and path to keep the practice vibrant.

Five-minute meditation. Stopping to do a mini meditation can also give you some relaxation benefits.

- Find a quiet, calming environment.
- Set a clock or timer for five minutes so you don't worry about time.
- Sit erect on the floor or a chair; try not to strain your back—a comfortable posture is important. If you're sitting on the floor, sit in a cross-legged position. If you're on a chair, place both feet flat on the ground in front of you. Place your palms on your knees or thighs. Try to keep your shoulders level and your hips aligned with your spine.
- Focus your gaze downward or some distance in front of you or close your eyes.
- Take slow, deep breaths. These breaths should feel easy and natural, not forced. Focus on the in-and-out motion of your breath through your nose and the rise and fall of your abdomen.
- Concentrate on your muscles, relaxing them as you think about them, and releasing their tension as you exhale.
- Try to avoid letting your thoughts stray from your own posture, breathing, and relaxation. As thoughts enter your mind, let them float away. Enjoy the state of relaxation and try to keep this feeling with you throughout the day.

Laughing meditation. Don't laugh, but studies consistently demonstrate that laughing is a very healthy form of exercise and has hormone-balancing effects. It is also a mind-body experience. Laughter represents a willingness to project your emotions rather than suppress them. In busy and stressful times, it's easy to forget to giggle. Try to laugh together as a couple, whether it's through a game of tickle, watching a funny movie, or reminiscing about funny times. When you're in the throes of laughter, try to extend it, keep it going, and basically milk it for what you can. There's an exercise that some people find helpful, though it might not be for everyone. There are

ACUPUNCTURE TO RELIEVE STRESS

Acupuncture is an ancient Chinese medicine practice that has become one of the most popular complementary therapies in this country. There's a growing body of research supporting its use in relieving stress. The practitioner places needles in specific points along *meridians* in order to free up energy, or *chi*. Acupuncture has been shown to promote the release of neurotransmitters such as pain-relieving endorphins. Studies of its effect on the stress reaction suggest that it can even reduce activity of the sympathetic nervous system. Some studies have also found that it can improve success rates during fertility treatments (more about that in the treatment section; see page 229). For referrals, visit the website of the National Certification Commission for Acupuncture and Oriental Medicine (www.nccaom.org). If you want to try it out, make sure that you're seeing a licensed acupuncturist. If your practitioner recommends any herbal treatments along with your procedure, discuss it with your fertility specialist first, as most herbs act as BioUnknowns and can trigger a hormonal *imbalance* that can interfere with your ability to conceive.

three phases to this exercise, each of which should last between 5 and 15 minutes.

◆ Begin by loosening up. Stretch your facial muscles through slow deep breaths, yawning, and even making funny faces. Remember, it's all about laughter.

◆ Imagine a funny situation you've experienced or a scene from a comedy that you really enjoyed. As you begin to smile and laugh, take your thoughts to even further extremes of that situation to really get your laughter going. If you need help, have your partner tickle you—you'll both wind up laughing.

◆ Conclude through several minutes of quiet meditation. Sit quietly, eyes closed, and focus on taking slow and full deep breaths.

PRINCIPLE TWO: MONITOR YOUR SLEEP HABITS

Though your body is at rest, sleep is one of the most active times of day for your brain. During sleep, we consolidate memory, repair daily wear and tear to our bodies, recharge our immune function, recycle various neurotransmitters, produce key hormones, and coordinate reproductive functions. Studies show that more than 80 percent of women ovulate between midnight and 8 a.m., so sleep disruptions can have a direct impact on your fertility.

There is no universal sleep requirement, as we all need different amounts of sleep. Take the following sleep questionnaire to see if you're getting enough sleep—not everyone needs eight hours. You should awake in the morning feeling refreshed and have adequate daytime energy to function at your best.

SLEEP RISK ASSESSMENT*

Use the following ratings to assess your risk of falling asleep during the following activities.

>   0 — Fully alert, no chance of falling asleep
>   1 — Might fall asleep
>   2 — I'm fighting to stay awake
>   3 — It's pretty likely that I will fall asleep

If I were . . .   My Chance of Falling Asleep Is . . .

1. Talking to partner   _____

2. Driving for 30 minutes in the early afternoon   _____

3. Attending a meeting in the evening   _____

4. Reading this book in the afternoon   _____

5. Waiting in the car for my partner   _____

6. Watching a movie in a dark theatre   _____

7 In the waiting room before an MD visit   _____

8. Getting a massage at my favorite spa   _____

9. On a short (1- to 2-hour) plane or train ride   _____

10. Driving for an hour around sunset   _____

                                          TOTAL: _____

Total your score. Here's the bottom line:

0–9: You're meeting your sleep needs.
10–12: You're pushing yourself a bit too hard.
13–20: You need more sleep.
21–30: Without more sleep, you're at risk of injury.

*Modified from the Epworth Sleepiness Scale

YOUR CIRCADIAN RHYTHM AND YOUR FERTILITY

One of the most damaging aspects of prolonged stress is how it affects your sleep and your circadian rhythms, the daily shifts your body makes. Disruptions in these cycles can directly affect your fertility. Your body functions in shifts, with many functions coming to life in the morning and certain jobs relegated to the night shift, when you're in your deepest sleep. These shifts are regulated by your brain's *suprachiasmatic nucleus,* or *SCN.* If your SCN senses that these shifts are disrupted, say, by not sleeping well, your circadian rhythms will be thrown off, disturbing many of the functions that normally occur at night. We know that poor sleep can affect your fertility in at least four ways.

- Poor sleep can prevent ovulation, which occurs in the middle of the night; women who work the night shift have a higher risk of ovulatory problems.
- Poor sleep keeps stress hormones elevated—under normal conditions, your body would reset your stress hormones to baseline levels while you're in your deepest sleep.
- People who don't sleep well have a higher incidence of obesity.
- Poor sleep contributes to insulin resistance, which can lower fertility.

If you're not sleeping well or feel overly tired during the day, consider the following troubleshooting tips.

Eat right. To get more daytime energy, eat more protein rich foods in the morning. To ease into a nighttime lull, eat more Power Carbs at night. A high-protein meal at night can boost your body temperature, interfering with your daily temperature fluctuation and lightening your sleep. Avoid caffeine at least seven hours before your normal bedtime.

Boost your melatonin production. Your SCN, the commander of your circadian rhythms, is located just behind your eyes and activated by light. As the sun rises, the SCN wakes up your morning hormonal shifts. But as the sun sets, the diminished light activates your brain's *pineal gland,* which secretes melatonin. A key function of melatonin is to keep the SCN dormant—and you sleepy—until the morning light peaks in.

To boost melatonin—and improve your sleep—try to eat foods containing the amino acid *tryptophan,* one of the key building blocks of melatonin. These include (from highest to lowest sources) spinach,

Did you know ?

A group of at least 10 genes in your DNA, collectively called *clock genes,* regulate your circadian rhythm in each cell of your body, giving your cells a sense of time. Clock genes provide a general guide for cells to coordinate with one another, but they can't adjust to seasonal changes in the length of the day nor to travel across time zones. Therefore, we rely on our hormones to reset and synchronize cellular function each day. In fact, hormones give your brain the ability to override these genes during times of stress, starvation, onset of puberty, or other situations that aren't accounted for by their genetic code.

seaweed, peanuts with skin, sesame seeds, tofu, mushrooms, lentils, and bananas. By the way, though turkey contains tryptophan, eating it doesn't increase the concentration of tryptophan in the brain. The amino acid is best absorbed when eaten as part of a Power Carb meal, and will have the greatest effect on sleep if eaten at dinner.

Develop good bedtime habits. Our brains adjust to behavioral patterns and our hormones shift in anticipation of regular daily events, so try to go to sleep and wake up at the same time every day. Other helpful tips for a good night's sleep include restricting daytime napping to 30 minutes or less, moving your alarm clock away from your bed so the time doesn't serve as a distraction, not staying in bed more than 15 to 30 minutes if you're awake, and keeping your bedroom dark and cool. If you have insomnia, only use your bed for sleep and sex, not for reading or watching TV.

Avoid sleep supplements. Although many supplements are sold as "natural sleep aids," most of them haven't been studied and may contain additional ingredients or might trigger hormonal imbalance. While you're trying to conceive, I recommend that you avoid them to minimize your risk.

Treat insomnia when necessary. If you can't get the rest you need, I recommend that you discuss the occasional use of a prescription sleep aid with your health care provider. I think the best available option is a BioSimilar hormone called Rozerem. It works the same way as the melatonin your body naturally produces to foster sleep, but does so throughout the night—a distinct advantage over the supplement forms of melatonin, which lose their effectiveness partway through the night and can create a rebound insomnia at around four o'clock in the morning. These supplements may also have a negative impact on ovulation. Rozerem is not habit forming and, unlike other sleep aids, does not produce rebound insomnia when you stop using it. It does not interfere with ovulation.

PRINCIPLE THREE: SUPPORT EACH OTHER

Infertility can place tremendous stress on a couple. Psychologists who work with infertility couples notice that men and women do not respond to infertility in the same way, nor at the same time. Typically, the woman is more devastated and wants to move into treatments faster than her partner. She also wants him to feel similarly and can be disappointed with him because he's not experiencing the same level of sadness or anxiety. The man more often wants to take a wait-and-see approach and wants his partner to stop obsessing about it. Men also tend to feel like they have to be emotionally strong, and avoid expressing their own feelings of disappointment or grief. It's important to understand these tendencies and the different styles of coping that may be at work in your relationship. This is a time to learn to listen to each other's feelings and be as supportive and understanding as possible.

Here are some of the top stressors that you or your partner may be experiencing.

Feeling helpless. Fertility can contribute to a sense of loss of control over your life and your body. Educating yourself about your options and participating in the decision making can help you feel in control, not powerless. This is among some of the most compelling reasons for reading this book and becoming your own advocate.

> ### Did you know ?
>
> Men and women wake with the highest testosterone levels of the day, providing an early morning boost in libido and promoting morning sexual activity. That was before our modern workday squeezed this pleasure out of the morning. Some experts theorize that the lengthening of our workday and our longer commutes have contributed to our falling fertility rate.

Lack of intimacy. With timed sex, your sex life can easily start to feel clinical and less romantic. Men can often feel that the only reason

THE HORMONE PLAYER

Oxytocin is released during labor and orgasm. It's considered a bonding hormone, able to cement intimate relationships and trigger your brain to recognize that the tension of the orgasm has passed. A hug or reassuring pat on the back can trigger small amounts of this hormone to be released and significantly lower stress levels.

their wives want to make love is to extract sperm from them. To minimize these feelings, try to have sex outside of your fertile window, too. Be extra sensitive to these issues, and be open to discussing your feelings. The more creative you can be during sex, the less clinical it will feel.

Fertility 24-7. For people going through fertility treatment, fertility can become the only thing they talk about. Try to reserve *fertility-free* times, when you agree not to talk about your desire to have children or your fertility progress.

Financial pressure. Financial concerns can be a major source of stress in couples—treatments can be expensive and are often not covered by insurance. It's common for couples to disagree on how much of their savings to spend or how much to borrow in their quest to become pregnant. Try to discuss these issues in advance—what your cap might be (you can change it down the road if the situation changes). This book will help you minimize your costs by avoiding unnecessary tests and treatments.

"Well-meaning" comments. Family and friends might badger you with questions about when you plan to start your family, or you may be subjected to well-meaning but unhelpful comments such as "if it's meant to be, it'll happen." Many women begin avoiding social situations because they feel that the emotional pain of seeing pregnant women or newborn babies is too great. Men may experience this as well. Sit down together and explore your feelings about whether to discuss your fertility problems with others (and with whom) or keep them private. Consider how much information you want to reveal. You may want to script a response you can both use that protects your privacy and emotions. Give yourselves permission to avoid

social situations that might be too uncomfortable. And if you see your partner beginning to squirm in a social situation, take the cue and make a graceful exit.

Disrupted lifestyle. Treatment can interfere with work and vacations, and may even begin to feel like a full-time job. Many people begin to put their lives on hold during treatment, postponing vacations or plans to switch jobs. If this happens to you, consider taking some time off of active treatment for a month or two. Go on a few day or weekend trips; even work in a vacation if possible. Use the time to reconnect with one another and take a breather from the pressure.

Not enough support. Consider reaching out to a support group with a philosophy shared by you and your partner. These are a few national organizations, but you might be able to find local groups through Internet groups, your physicians, or local civic associations.

> **Did you know ?**
>
> New research has found that when relationship stress develops within a couple—a frequent occurrence among infertility patients—more aggressive medical treatment is often required.

- *RESOLVE* is a nationwide infertility education and support association with regional networks. To find a chapter near you, check its website at www.resolve.org.
- The *American Fertility Association* (www.theafa.org) is a patient advocacy and education group offering support groups nationwide.
- *Fertile Hope* (www.fertilehope.org) is a nonprofit organization dedicated to helping cancer patients who are facing infertility.

PRINCIPLE FOUR: JOURNALING FOR STRESS REDUCTION

Journaling is one of the most effective tools for managing emotions and relieving stress. Writing is more powerful than talking because it calls for more introspection, and it helps you carefully identify your feelings and reactions. Many people have reported that journaling brings physical benefits along with emotional relief. Studies show that by journaling regularly, your words begin to reflect a greater sense of optimism, your memory improves, you become more effective in your daily activities, and you're less bothered by intrusive thoughts. Try to spend at least 15 minutes writing every day—especially in times of greater stress. If you're new to journaling and aren't sure what to write about, try *freewriting*, which entails writing continuously to fill a page, without stopping. Write whatever comes to mind, even if it doesn't make sense. Here's an example of one of my patient's freewriting.

JENNY'S FREEWRITING

I'm so frustrated and don't even know where to begin or what to say. There are so many thoughts swirling around in my head, why this is happening to me, why didn't I realize I had a problem sooner. It's so depressing and so ironic, all those years on birth control. And the panic when my period was late four years ago because we weren't "ready yet." I don't know what to say, but I'll just keep writing and hope that something coherent comes out. It all started when Steve's sister started talking about having kids and we all began to fantasize about holidays, birthday parties, and family vacations. We thought it would be so fun for our kids to be around the same age. Now she's pregnant with number two (grr) and we have nothing. I think I first knew in my gut there was a problem after the third month of trying. It was just a feeling or maybe a fear, probably a fear. I heard stories about infertility, so it's there in the back of your mind. But that sort of thing only happens to other people . . . right? I tried not to think of it as a problem for a while, which is why we waited so long to get help. I probably didn't want to acknowledge there was a problem or whatever. I lost my train of thought, and I'd rather not go there because it makes me feel guilty, like we'd already have a child by now if we hadn't waited. But Steve waited too, he's always hoped we'd conceive naturally in the heat of passion. I guess we were both in denial. But I wish he had taken my initial concerns more seriously. If he showed he was worried about it too, we probably would have acted sooner. But he dismissed it so I did too. Not that I'm blaming him but I hate when I don't listen to my gut. It keeps happening and always gets me in trouble, but now I'm off the topic. What else should I write?

When you become more comfortable with journaling, try to find the words that most accurately describe your deepest feelings surrounding the event or emotions you're writing about. If nothing has happened that had an emotional impact on you since your last journal entry, write about something that happened in the past that still upsets you. Describe how you felt about it then and now. Write about what you may have learned from a particular experience or what you could have done differently. This will help you prevent the helpless feeling that can contribute to chronic stress.

◆　　◆　　◆

Reducing stress is the third and last part of my program to improve your hormone balance. In the next chapter, I'll provide information about what steps you can take while you're mastering this program in order to improve your chances of fertility at home, and how to prepare for your first consultation if you decide to consider fertility treatments.

7
Your First Steps to Pregnancy Start at Home

It can take three to four months of following my program to fully reap its hormone-balancing effects and increase your chance of becoming pregnant, but this doesn't have to be a holding period. I am certain that some of you will get pregnant during this time without pursuing any fertility treatment. But as you're adopting the program, you can also take the first steps toward treating your fertility. These include tracking your ovulation and "timing" sex to your peak fertility window, as well as gathering information to prepare for your first fertility consultation so that you're as knowledgeable as possible about your personal fertility issues (or, as fertility specialists say, your *fertility factors*). This can help you avoid unnecessary tests and make your fertility treatment more focused, so that you don't waste precious time, energy, and money.

YOUR MENSTRUAL CYCLES

Many women don't pay much attention to when their menstrual cycles occur or if they've changed over the months or years. That's especially true for women who've been taking a birth control pill. However, as I often say, "symptoms matter," and there is no more obvious sign of changes in your hormones than your menstrual cycles. Understanding

JUMP-START YOUR FERTILITY EVALUATION . . . AT HOME!

I've found that many couples are anxious to know their fertility status, and are too impatient to delay their appointment for three to six months as they establish hormone balance through the Perfect Balance Fertility Program. Now there's a very effective way to get a basic read on your fertility factors before you see a specialist. Fertell, the first home fertility test, became available in 2007. This test will help you determine whether you should move rapidly to seek a complete fertility evaluation. If your test results are normal, you are more likely to get pregnant by following my program and the guidelines in this chapter. If the test is abnormal, refer to Part 3 and start the process of seeking a more thorough assessment of your fertility factors while continuing with my program. If a man has an abnormal result, it means his sperm are contributing to the fertility problem. If a woman tests positive, her ovaries are contributing. The test is considered accurate in 95 percent of couples tested. It is FDA approved and costs about $100. I strongly recommend this test. Visit www.fertell.com for more information.

them can help predict your chance of conception and provide insights into your fertility problem.

The most important characteristics are the length of your cycles and their variation from month to month. Regular cycles, averaging 27 to 29 days, are a sign of peak fertility. One study of couples with difficulties conceiving found that women whose cycles were regular and averaged 29 days had the highest conception rate without treatment. If your cycles are longer than 39 days, consider seeing a fertility specialist in three months, rather than continue trying on your own. Balancing your hormones alone may not be enough to overcome your problem.

Start tracking your cycles in a fertility calendar, like the one in Appendix A, indicating which days bleeding starts and stops, and whether the flow was light, moderate, or heavy. Make notes of any other symptoms you have like cramps or spotting between periods. Write down when they occurred and their severity. Symptoms like headache or mood changes may also provide insight, especially if they recur with regularity.

DOCUMENTING YOUR FERTILE WINDOW

Having sex during the one to two days when you're most fertile is the best step you can take toward improving your chances of conceiving.

Although the average monthly pregnancy rate for sexually active couples is around 18 percent, studies show that when women use an accurate method to predict ovulation, fertility rates approach 50 percent.

You are most fertile the day of and the day prior to the day you ovulate. An egg will only be fertile for about a day after its release, so it's critical that healthy sperm are either in the fallopian tube waiting for the egg or arrive shortly after ovulation occurs.

Try to time sex to the two days before ovulation preceded by two days of abstinence. Use the Clearblue Easy Fertility Monitor (www.clearblueeasy.com) to get advance warning of when you ovulate. This monitor tracks when luteinizing hormone (LH) peaks in your urine, giving you 24 to 36 hours notice before ovulation. It also measures a rise in estrogen, which can give you at least one extra day of advance notice. A 2007 study demonstrated that the Clearblue monitor nearly doubled the pregnancy rate during the first couple of months it was used, even in couples that had been trying to conceive for up to two years.

MAKE IT A "DATE NIGHT"

Some couples mourn the loss of the joy and spontaneity of sex when it has to be scheduled to optimize fertility. I suggest you turn it into a two-day affair during your most fertile period. If possible, have sex both nights to take advantage of the fertile window. The key to making it not feel like an "appointment" is, in a word, seduction. Clear time on your schedule, make a romantic dinner, or plan to eat out. Keep it romantic, putting any issues or stress-button topics on the back burner. Since it may require a shift in your approach to sex, remind each other, if necessary, that some extra effort in the seduction phase may be needed.

Monitoring hormones secreted in the urine does not always give you the exact day of ovulation. It is often combined with methods that track changes in your physiology that occur during your fertile window, such as basal body temperature charting—measuring your early morning temperature—and monitoring cervical mucus. Another approach I recommend is using a high-tech tool like the OV-Watch (www.ovwatch.com), a wrist computer containing an advanced biosensor that monitors the amount of chloride—half of the molecule that makes up ordinary table salt—for its peak level. Chloride peaks several days before ovulation

Case in Point

Paul and Jane were married shortly before he was shipped out for military service. Since his tour of duty kept being extended, they had spent little time together in the three years they had been married, and they were becoming impatient to begin a family—they wanted to have three children together. Jane, 30, came to see me to discuss how to time her fertile window to his leaves and possibly store sperm as a backup plan, so she could become pregnant while he was away, a plan they both had agreed on.

Paul, 45, had fathered two children with his previous partner. But Jane had never been pregnant. She had always taken birth control pills, which she started in her teens to lighten her heavy menstrual cycles. Jane had a history of elevated cholesterol and high blood pressure, but wasn't taking any medications for these conditions. Paul was not scheduled to be on leave for another six months. I instructed Jane to stop the birth control pill and begin using an ovulation kit for the next four months in order to establish her fertility. She also began the Perfect Balance program with the goal of losing 10 pounds and improving her cholesterol and blood pressure. Four months later, she had lost 12 pounds and appeared to be ovulating normally. Next, we tried to reset her menstrual cycle to coincide with Paul's leave. I had Jane restart a birth control pill and then stop it one week before his return home. It worked like a charm. On his first leave, she got pregnant.

(causing the bloating you may experience) in response to shifts in your levels of estradiol. The watch is worn for at least six hours each night during sleep, beginning no later than the third day of your menstrual cycle. It's easy to use and gives you a little more advance notice than other fertility monitors—meaning more time to plan for sex.

SEX AND FERTILITY

I've probably heard every myth about the relationship between sex and fertility ever spoken. Because I know my patients hear about the benefits of certain positions, abstinence, and even whether having an orgasm can harm or help their efforts to conceive, I try to do some myth busting up front so my patients don't have to ask questions that they find embarrassing. I've been amazed by some of the instructions patients were given by friends, family, or advice columnists. Here's what I tell my patients:

WHEN TO SEE A SPECIALIST

Some couples wait too long before seeking treatment, while others jump in too quickly. The standard recommendation is to try to conceive for 12 months if you're under 35 before seeking an evaluation, six months if you're 35 or over. These waiting periods are based on the average monthly pregnancy rate—80 to 90 percent of couples become pregnant within one year. But it's a generalization that doesn't consider a couple's individual fertility factors, or the age of the male, or how seriously you have been trying. For instance, it matters if you've been casually trying or using an ovulation detection method and precisely timing your sexual activity. It also depends on how you might want your children spaced and how many fertile years you have left. I recommend that if you've been following the Perfect Balance program for at least six months, and using an accurate method of ovulation prediction, it's time to seek a specialist. For women that aren't ovulating or are over 35 years of age, seek a consultation with a reproductive endocrinologist after only three months.

Your position during or after sex will not improve your fertility, despite what you may have heard about the benefits of standing on your head or keeping your legs in the air after sex. Sperm are unaffected by the forces of gravity. Rather than doing these mood-dampening calisthenics, indulge in postcoital intimacies to help strengthen your emotional bond.

Frequent sexual activity will not diminish your chances of conception. The only truth to this myth is that you should abstain from sex the two days before your peak fertility window—this window is two days before ovulation—but you can and should have frequent sex during your fertile window. There are a few rare situations in which men with a low sperm count might be instructed to schedule ejaculation around specific treatment days.

Having an orgasm probably doesn't help you conceive—at least it has not been validated through studies. But there is some rationale to the theory. During an orgasm, the vagina contracts, causing it to shorten by about 30 percent and causing the cervix to get nearer to the top of the vagina, where the man's sperm is deposited—theoretically creating an easy entry to the womb. Additionally, contractions within the uterus may enhance the entry of sperm and speed their

Fertility Fact

A Sperm-Safe Lubricant

Studies of infertility patients reveal that women are about twice as likely to experience pain during "timed sex" than spontaneous sex—largely because of decreased lubrication. Less lubrication can be a side effect of some fertility medications, but it can also be related to stress or anxiety or a lack of arousal caused by the clinical nature of scheduled sex. Many women have avoided popular lubricants because they've been shown to interfere with normal sperm function. There is at least one product, called Pre-Seed, that won't reduce fertility. Pre-Seed has the proper acid-to-base balance to protect sperm. (For more information, visit www.preseed.com.)

passage to the fallopian tubes. In reality, however, one out of three women report that they rarely achieve an orgasm. Of those that do have orgasms, less than half have one during intercourse. Clearly, two-thirds of women—the sum total of those who don't have orgasm during intercourse—do not have fertility issues. Having said that, your sexual satisfaction is important, and there are solutions to *anorgasmia*—the inability to achieve an orgasm. You may wish to seek a specialist to assist with a diagnosis and treatment. However, rest assured that this is not a critical fertility factor. If you experience pain or vaginal bleeding following intercourse, please see chapter 12 to consider whether you may have endometriosis. If your partner has an ejaculatory disorder such as premature ejaculation or erectile dysfunction, see chapter 8 on male factors.

BEING YOUR OWN FERTILITY ADVOCATE

Many couples choose to go no further than monitoring their ovulation and timing their sex in their quest to have a baby. By following the program, many of you will conceive without pursuing fertility treatments. But some do venture into the fertility-treatment world, and if you choose to move forward, it's best to proceed with as much knowledge about your fertility and your health as possible to get the most individualized treatment. To begin, I recommend that you gather information about your medical history in advance.

You can discuss this information with your OB, who can recommend the most appropriate tests. In fact, the information that I'll provide in

Part 3, "Understanding Your Fertility Factors," will give you and your partner enough knowledge about your conditions to be able to request specific tests and question any tests your doctor recommends that may seem inappropriate or outdated.

Your answers to the questionnaires on pages 124 and 125 will help you and your doctor determine which diagnostic tests you should consider, and help guide your treatment. Bring this list of questions with your answers to your consultation.

TIMING AND GENDER SELECTION

One of the enduring fertility myths is that you can increase your chance of having a boy or a girl if you time sex just right. This is loosely based on scientific data. Your baby's sex is determined by which sperm penetrates the egg: an X (female chromosome) or a Y (male chromosome). Studies have shown that Y-bearing sperm do swim a bit faster, but have a shorter life span after ejaculation. In theory, if you had sex at the time of ovulation, it would increase the chance of having a boy because the Y sperm would reach the egg the fastest, and if you had sex several days before ovulation you'd boost the chance for a female, because the female sperm will have outlived the males. However, when put to the test, these methods have failed. Other recommendations regarding your sexual position, men wearing boxers versus briefs, and timing sex to your vaginal pH have been scientifically tested and disproven. My real concern is that following some of these recommendations may hinder fertility by restricting sexual activity during your fertile window.

PREPARING TO SEE A FERTILITY SPECIALIST

Consider making an appointment to be seen in three, six, or nine months, depending on your situation. But whom should you see? This is one area you should research carefully. Going to the right doctor might speed your journey to pregnancy—and reduce the amount of unnecessary tests or ineffective treatments you'll receive. Keep this perspective in mind when doing your legwork: Research in the field of human reproduction has progressed at an astounding rate over the last two decades. In order to remain current with recommendations, a specialist must always keep abreast of the latest findings and revise his approach to treatment appropriately. This isn't possible for the typical

HEALTH HISTORY QUESTIONNAIRE FOR WOMEN

Medical history. This includes previous illnesses, ongoing medical conditions, and information that may affect your chance of success.

Did your mother take the medication DES when she was pregnant with you?　　Yes　No

Did you weigh less than 6 pounds at birth?　　Yes　No

Did you experience your first period before your 11th birthday
or much earlier than all your peers?　　Yes　No

Have you had two or more previous miscarriages?　　Yes　No

Have you had gonorrhea, chlamydia, or pelvic inflammatory disease (PID)?　　Yes　No

Have you tested positive for human papillomavirus (HPV)
or had a procedure to treat an abnormal Pap smear?　　Yes　No

Surgical history. The surgeries listed here are most often linked to infertility.

Have you ever had a tubal ligation ("tubes tied"), ectopic pregnancy
(the fetus started to grow in the fallopian tube), surgery to remove
your appendix, or surgery to treat PID?　　Yes　No

Have you had surgery for uterine fibroids?　　Yes　No

Have you had surgery for pelvic pain or endometriosis?　　Yes　No

Have you had surgery for ovarian cysts or had an ovary removed?　　Yes　No

Have you had more than one cesarean section or had an infection after
the delivery of your last child?　　Yes　No

Have you had multiple abortions or experienced an infection following a
dilation and curettage (D & C)?　　Yes　No

Social history. This can be awkward for many health care providers to discuss with you. It's easiest if you know what factors have the greatest impact on your chance to conceive so that you can actively direct your doctor. Focus on the following:

Have you been sexually active now or with previous partners for longer than
three years without the use of contraception, but never got pregnant?　　Yes　No

Do you experience pain during intercourse?　　Yes　No

Do you participate in marathons or other extreme sports?　　Yes　No

Do you lack a male partner or identify yourself as lesbian?　　Yes　No

Family history. Your issues with fertility may have a genetic component to it.

Did your mother experience difficulty conceiving or have more
than two miscarriages?　　Yes　No

Do you have a sister with infertility?   Yes   No

Has your mother or sister had endometriosis?   Yes   No

Has your mother or sister been diagnosed with or treated for uterine fibroids?   Yes   No

HEALTH HISTORY QUESTIONNAIRE FOR MEN

Medical history. These conditions may directly impact the quality of your sperm.

Have you had mumps or any illness with prolonged fevers above
104 degrees since puberty?   Yes   No

Have you experienced any trauma to the testicles or groin severe
enough to cause swelling or prolonged pain?   Yes   No

Are you taking medications for blood pressure, diabetes, epilepsy,
prostate problems, and impotence, or to prevent hair loss?   Yes   No

Surgical history. Discuss any surgery to your testicles or scrotum as well
as the following two procedures.

Have you had a hernia repair?   Yes   No

Have you had a vasectomy with or without a previous attempt at reversing it?   Yes   No

Social history. This includes aspects of your past that you may find embarrassing, but
being forthright about your history can save you considerable time and expense.

Have you been sexually active with your current or previous partner for
a year without the use of contraception, but never had a pregnancy?   Yes   No

Have you ever been exposed to toxic chemicals at work?   Yes   No

Are you regularly exposed to high heat from saunas or at work?   Yes   No

Do you participate in marathons or other extreme sports?   Yes   No

Are you taking any supplements to build muscle, improve sexual performance,
shrink prostate swelling, or reduce hair loss?   Yes   No

Family history. Your issues with fertility may have a genetic component to it.

Has your father or brother had a history of a low sperm count or infertility?   Yes   No

Do you have a brother with cystic fibrosis or have had nieces or nephews with
any birth defects?   Yes   No

SECONDARY INFERTILITY

Some couples who've already had a child might have trouble becoming pregnant again—a condition referred to as *secondary infertility*. It's often assumed that someone's fertility doesn't change, but this is far from the truth. If you're experiencing secondary infertility, you should make sure that you're evaluated thoroughly.

One common cause of secondary infertility is age. Fertility drops as you age, more dramatically and earlier for women than for men. Many changes also tend to occur with age that can upset your hormone balance and diminish fertility. The usual suspects: weight gain, a sedentary lifestyle, or the development of hormonal conditions like hypothyroidism or diabetes. Additionally, if you or your partner are on any medications or have been diagnosed with any other medical conditions since your last pregnancy, these factors may also be contributing.

Finally, there are various acquired but symptom-free problems that may cause a change in your fertility status, such as the formation of scar tissue from previous surgery (for example, a cesarean section for women or a hernia repair for men), the growth of uterine fibroids, or the development of endometriosis. Just because you've been pregnant before or think that you know what your greatest obstacle to becoming pregnant is, don't skip a complete evaluation before creating your treatment plan.

general care provider, or even many obstetricians. In order to find someone qualified and current in their knowledge, I recommend you check for a referral through the American Society for Reproductive Medicine (ASRM) at www.asrm.org.

The ASRM is a multidisciplinary organization of specialists involved in researching and treating all aspects of infertility. Its members include doctors, nurses, therapists, and laboratory technicians from fields as diverse as obstetrics and gynecology, endocrinology, urology, psychology, and embryology. Members are not all board-certified reproductive endocrinologists, but they have a specific interest in infertility and typically keep current on the latest fertility treatments. There are many qualified OBs who can run your first set of tests, but be sure yours is a member of ASRM, as there are also many underqualified OBs who add "fertility specialist" to their shingle without having any recent fertility training.

Some of you, on the other hand, will need more advanced treatments like IVF or may have very complicated problems. You should see a board-certified reproductive endocrinology and infertility subspecialist. To earn this designation, a physician has to complete a four year ob-gyn residency and then continue on for an additional two- or three-year fellowship focused on the study of reproductive hormones and fertility. To find a subspecialist in your community, visit the website of the Society for Reproductive Endocrinology and Infertility (www.socrei.org) and click on the "find members" link. You might also get referrals from friends or a local support group. Just be sure to ask if a referral is a member of ASRM.

If you've already begun working with a fertility center or are ready to choose one, refer to the conclusion for more details on what to look for in a center—qualifications, success rates, and personalities—and how to deal with them to get the treatments you need.

GETTING MENTALLY PREPARED FOR TREATMENT

Many couples with fertility issues end up feeling as if they're being shuttled from one treatment to the next, with the events getting beyond their control and desires. Feeling this loss of control can lead to depression and stress and can negatively affect your relationship. In some countries, couples are required to get counseling before receiving fertility treatment. Although I routinely recommend that my patients meet with a therapist, I realize that the cost and time of therapy make it impractical for some patients. As an alternative, I recommend taking a self-efficacy questionnaire (see page 128) to determine how likely you are to make choices that are right for you, rather than being pushed in one direction or another by doctors, well meaning parents and in-laws, and even each other. This test can help predict if you are at risk of suffering significant stress or depression, and if you would benefit greatly from emotional support.

WRITE A FERTILITY PLAN

Some of the decisions you will make in your effort to have a baby demand that you look deeply inside yourselves. The choices you'll face can call up questions about your religious values, your morals and

FERTILITY SELF-EFFICACY QUESTIONNAIRE

I recommend that you and your partner take this test now and repeat it at least every two to three months as you pursue pregnancy. Write your scores down in a journal so you can track them and monitor whether they're getting worse or improving.

	Never		Sometimes		Always
	1	2	3	4	5

1. I'm an optimistic person.

2. I enjoy being around pregnant women.

3. I'm happy when I learn of someone else's pregnancy.

4. I enjoy my sexual relationship.

5. I am happy and easily able to laugh.

6. I am confident that I will become pregnant.

7. I can handle mood fluctuations.

8. I am able to keep negative feelings about infertility in perspective.

9. I am maintaining my normal responsibilities and routines.

10. I can cope with questions from family and friends.

11. I feel good about my relationship.

12. I believe that I am doing my best to reach my goals.

13. I can deal with discouragement.

14. I can share in the joy of others.

15. I don't blame myself or my partner.

Total your score. Here's the bottom line:

If you have a score below 45 or find that over time your score is dropping, you would benefit from the support of a trained therapist. This is somewhat subjective, so you need to decide if you're satisfied with your scores, even if they're higher or if you feel you would benefit from help. By comparing scores with your partner, you can also determine your ability to support each other through fertility treatment. See Appendix F for a list of organizations that offer referrals to therapists.

ethics, how important it is for you to have a genetic legacy, and your financial situation. Before seeing a specialist, you and your partner should discuss these issues. The decisions you make now will help guide you through the options you'll face later. I recommend you create a *fertility plan*—an idealized blueprint of your goals and comfort levels in your quest to create a family. Answer a series of questions (see Appendix D, "Fertility Plan"). For instance, are you willing to go through IVF? How do you feel about having a multiple pregnancy? Are you open to using donated sperm or eggs? What would you do if you became pregnant with triplets or more?

I recommend that you start looking at these questions now. You may not understand all the terminology or options yet, but you'll learn more about your fertility factors and your treatment options as you progress through the book. Remember, none of these questions has an answer that is right or wrong. Instead, they're based upon your personal beliefs and preferences. And, of course, you can always reconsider and modify your plan. It might also help you to identify potential areas of conflict between you and your partner before you're asked these questions by a health care provider. If you and your partner are at an impasse regarding any of the questions, skip it for now—it might not ever come up for you and if it seems necessary later, you can revisit it. By preparing ahead of time, you'll be able to avoid answering these questions on the spot, minimize your stress later, and be in control of your own fertility.

3

Understanding Your Fertility Factors

Introduction:
Getting the Right Diagnosis

If you are thinking of pursuing fertility treatment or even if you have already had an evaluation and started treatment, I urge you to read this section to gain a thorough understanding of what fertility factors might be obstacles to you as a couple. You will have the greatest chance of becoming pregnant if you can guide your health care provider to individualize your treatment to meet your needs. With the growing success of fertility clinics, many diagnostic tests and many treatments tend to be driven by *protocols*—predetermined sets of tests and procedures that are given to all patients. That means that you might get tests that you don't need, and might not be offered tests that you do need. I firmly believe that the more actively involved you are in understanding the evaluation process and the fertility factors involved in your reproductive health, the greater your chance of success will be—and the faster it will come.

There are two scenarios that you might fall into, and in both cases, you'll be far better off by being educated about your factors. The first is the most common: the majority of couples facing infertility in the United States will not see a fertility specialist for treatment, but will see an obstetrician instead. The reason for this is that there are only about 700 board-certified reproductive endocrinologists nationwide, and people living in many areas of the country don't have access to them. In addition, many obstetricians are now marketing themselves as specialists in fertility and attracting many fertility patients, yet many aren't able to stay up to date on the fertility research and may recommend tests that are not in your best interest or are even outdated. In some situations, there may even be an incentive to use these tests to generate income for doctors. The information in this section will help you feel emboldened to question any health care provider who is a nonspecialist. A competent provider will respond positively to your questions and concerns, and you will quickly develop a partnership with him or her as you proceed through your fertility testing and treatments.

If you find yourself in the second scenario, in which you are seeing qualified reproductive endocrinologists at a fertility center, you may have to be assertive about the tests they recommend. One of the major criticisms of these centers is that they tend to figure out what works for them, and apply that protocol to all of their patients. In order to receive individualized care that will help you rise above their established success rates, and avoid unnecessary tests and procedures, take the time to learn about your own fertility factors.

One last reason to know your own fertility factors is to lower your chances of being misdiagnosed with *unexplained infertility*—a designation given to one out of three couples that have undergone fertility testing. With this diagnosis, treatment will likely start at the most basic level, say, taking the hormone Clomid to stimulate egg production, and if that doesn't work (sometimes after numerous cycles), you'll climb your way up to IVF and beyond. There are many problems with this approach, but perhaps the biggest is that it wastes your precious time, money, and emotional resources. Though there is some uncertainty in reproductive medicine, a great deal of reliable information can be obtained with a thorough yet sensible evaluation.

The truth is, most fertility problems involve several contributing factors. Over the course of my career, I've come to fully appreciate the whole-body approach—or the whole-couple approach, to be more precise. But in following this approach, it's essential to be able to understand how much each fertility factor is contributing to the bigger infertility picture, rather than focus on only one aspect of what it takes to become pregnant. I developed a system of grading a couple's fertility factors so that I could gauge how mild or severe each factor is and whether it needs to be addressed in the couple's treatment. The main fertility factors that all specialists use are male factor, ovarian factor, tubal factor, and uterine factor. For each of these factors, I categorize you and your partner as factor 1 (presumed fertile), factor 2 (mild), factor 3 (moderate), factor 4 (severe). These designations are not set in stone. If you undergo treatments that are unsuccessful, you may need to revise your assessment based upon how you responded to the treatments. This is important, too, because even when a treatment is unsuccessful, you can come away with valuable information that will help you to consider what to do next. Each step on your journey counts.

In this section, I will take you step-by-step through each of the fertility factors that impact your reproductive health. Each chapter focuses on a different aspect of your or your partner's anatomy. I will first describe normal functioning, and then discuss any signs of problems, as well as your risk of having a particular fertility factor based on your medical and personal history. I will help you determine your fertility factor levels—often with the assistance of at-home questionnaires or diagnostic tests your doctor needs to order. As you read through the chapters, you'll see that you may need diagnostic tests to move forward, and you'll have to consult with either your obstetrician or a fertility specialist to request these before you can fully determine your factors. Though I have talked a lot about the cost of testing, I am in no way against testing. But I want you to get the most accurate, appropriate and cost-effective tests, and the ones that are going to yield the most useful information. If you need an ultrasound to visualize your ovaries, for example, I want you to request that your doctor use that opportunity to also visualize your uterus, rather than having separate tests that generate separate charges.

THE ULTRA ULTRASOUND

One of my favorite shortcuts to diagnosing fertility factors is a carefully timed hydrosonography (also known as a sonohysterogram), a type of ultrasound. This single exam can simultaneously estimate your ovarian factor, your uterine factor, and your tubal factor (the health of your fallopian tubes). It involves undergoing a pelvic ultrasound during the first half of your menstrual cycle. This test can reduce or eliminate your need for several other tests.

A word of caution here: certain diagnostic evaluations may not be covered by your insurance carrier or might not be available if you live in a rural area. In some cases, it may be worth the out-of-pocket expense of getting a more comprehensive examination that isn't covered, rather than wasting time getting one of the tests that I describe as unhelpful, even though your doctor recommended it and it is covered by insurance. Talk to your doctor about the cost and benefits of the tests she suggests.

I'm fully aware that I'm providing you with a lot of information—all of the latest information that's available. I have found, in general, that my fertility patients are starving for information, but I urge you to only take on what you can. You may feel like skipping over some details of a diagnostic test for a particular factor, and returning to it later if you're faced specifically with that issue.

One last note for those of you who know you have to turn to surrogates or donors: I urge you to read this entire section as well, since it will help you when choosing your donors. You'll learn about the factors that can affect the health of an egg or a sperm, or even the ability of a surrogate to successfully carry a pregnancy. Sometimes choosing a donor is based on emotional connections you might feel, but to give your future baby the greatest start, it's important to consider things like the age of the egg donor as well as her family and medical history.

HOW TO TALK TO YOUR DOCTORS

When you go for your consultation, bring a copy of both of your medical records from primary care physicians and ob-gyn. Be sure to review your records beforehand and flag anything with a Post-it that you think is incorrect. You should also bring your checklist of screening tests from chapter 3, and your answers to the questionnaires in chapter 7. In addition, bring what you learn in Part Three about your fertility factors, as well as what tests you believe you should have and feel most comfortable getting. I recommend that you summarize what you feel are the most relevant points in your history in a page or less. It should also include information about symptoms that you've noted as you've worked on restoring hormone balance. You will be surprised at how valuable this information is and how easily it could otherwise be overlooked.

Although your doctor will be very familiar with fertility factors, she may not be familiar with the system of factor *levels* that I have developed, because most centers do not have a tool like this that summarizes the severity of each facet of a couple's fertility. But a competent physician will understand the rationale of this objective approach. Your doctor might disagree with your suggestions and requests, and that's OK. You should be open to her opinions and expertise. Ideally, you should work in partnership with her.

Getting through your evaluation shouldn't be an intimidating process, but rather an enlightening one. By knowing what to expect and being able to anticipate the next step, your stress hormone levels will naturally lower and your success rate will rise. After you've completed your evaluation, you and your partner will be able to proceed to Part Four, "Your Fertility Plan: Making it Happen." Armed with this knowledge and confidence, you'll be able to finalize your fertility plan and move as quickly as possible toward your goal of giving birth to a child.

8 Male Factor

For at least one of every five couples unable to conceive, their infertility is linked exclusively to a male factor—either having too few sperm, sperm that don't function properly, or functional problems that prevent sperm from traveling through the male's reproductive system. For two of the four remaining couples, a male factor contributes to the couple's difficulty. Taken together, the male factor contributes to at least half of all fertility problems. Yet, men typically don't have obvious signals of reduced fertility comparable to the irregularity of a woman's menstrual cycle. That's why every couple evaluated at a fertility clinic

---

THE HORMONE PLAYERS

♦ **Testosterone** is the dominant sex hormone in men because it's present in such high amounts, and plays a critical role in sperm development.

♦ **Follicle-stimulating hormone (FSH)** provides a steady daily signal to the testicles to continue producing sperm, while in women, FSH levels shift throughout the monthly cycle.

♦ **Luteinizing hormone (LH)** promotes the continuous production of testosterone by the testicles.

♦ **Gonadotropin-releasing hormone (GnRH),** produced by the hypothalamus, triggers the pituitary gland to release these levels of FSH and LH.

Male Reproductive System

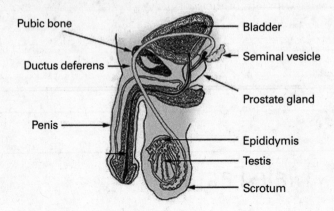

has to undergo an assessment of the male partner—even if he's fathered children before.

Typically, at the age of 11 or 12, a boy's hormones begin to kick in, but he won't begin producing sperm for another year or two. Specifically, his brain's hypothalamus starts releasing large pulses of GnRH, which signal the pituitary gland to release bursts of FSH and LH into the bloodstream. These hormones signal his body to begin producing immature sperm cells called *spermatogonia*. Once this process is initiated, it will typically continue for the rest of a male's life—preserving his potential fertility well into his 80s.

The pulses of FSH trigger the spermatogonia to begin a 90-day process of maturation called *spermatogenesis*—which entails the sperm cell dropping one copy of each chromosome so it can unite with the egg. The sperm also becomes more compact and grows a tail to propel itself toward an egg-in-waiting. The LH pulses trigger the sperm's helper cells, called *Leydig cells,* to produce testosterone.

The sperm mature within the testicles, specifically inside a network of pipes called the *seminiferous tubules*. Within the tubules, waves of sperm, called generations, move through six stages of development in sync with each other. Each tubule contains Sertoli and Leydig cells that help the developing sperm in different ways. The Sertoli cells protect a man's sperm from his own immune system, which views sperm as foreign cells (they have subtle genetic differences from other cells in his body). Leydig cells produce testosterone and other hormones that stim-ulate the development of the sperm.

Mature sperm ultimately migrate to the *epididymis,* a tightly coiled tube that sperm traverse in about four days before they empty into the *vas deferens.* There, sperm are transported to the *ejaculatory ducts,* where, during orgasm, they are forced out of the penis.

Since men produce sperm continuously, at any given moment, they have millions of sperm stored at various stages of development. But during the 90-day maturation process, the sperm are susceptible to dam-age created by hormone imbalances. So within the vast pool of sperm, only a small percentage—sometimes as low 15 percent in a "normal" specimen—are free of genetic and structural problems and are of high-enough quality to penetrate and fertilize an egg.

SEMEN ANALYSIS

If you are experiencing infertility, the first test you should get is a semen analysis, a basic assessment of your ejaculate. The test determines how many sperm are present, how motile (good at swimming) they are, and whether they show signs of being func-tionally impaired. These are the three main factors affecting male fertility. In this test, a man has to provide a semen sample to the clinic or a lab, and then the sample is carefully examined through a microscope or a computerized analyzer. This is not a perfect test, but it's the best tool we have.

Did you know ?

If your semen analysis is normal, it's extremely unlikely that a hormonal imbalance is causing male factor infertility.

A normal test confirms that sperm production is adequate, that all the tubes are unobstructed (or *patent*) and that a man can ejaculate an adequate number of sperm. However, it does not confirm that the sperm are fully functional and are able to fertilize an egg. In other words, your chance of having a possible male factor is markedly reduced, but not eliminated. Still, it provides enough information to help you decide on a course of treatment.

To perform a proper analysis, technicians look at millions of sperm through a microscope, and try to make generalizations about their quantity, size, and shape. This can make it somewhat subjective; several

Partner Pointer

Avoid Expensive Semen Tests

In the last decade, a number of sophisticated and expensive tests have been developed for semen analysis—antibody tests, blood tests, hormone tests, sperm penetration assays, and others. But for most men, none of these tests are necessary. In fact, some tests can be misleading and result in expensive and unnecessary treatments. The most basic semen analysis is all you'll need, saving you the time, expense, and the inconvenience of these new tests.

studies have found that when the same semen samples are shown to different laboratory technicians, the results were not always the same. Many big fertility centers have improved their results by using computer-assisted semen analysis (CASA), providing accurate counts, more detailed motility, and more precise evaluation of the size and shape of sperm. But if you're being seen by a small practice, an obstetrician, or a general practitioner, you'll probably be required to bring your specimen to a pathology lab. Most labs, however, don't use CASA.

INTERPRETING YOUR OWN SEMEN ANALYSIS

I believe it's important that you understand and are able to interpret your semen analysis and have access to the numbers. I've had patients tell me that their doctor simply told them their analysis "looks good" or "could be better," but this doesn't provide enough information to make an educated decision. Moreover, in some cases, doctors interpret an abnormal result as a zero chance of getting pregnant. But as long as sperm are present and moving, you have a slight chance of pregnancy.

Below I describe what you need to know about your semen analysis— what it tests for and how to interpret the results in order to help you understand to what degree your male factor is affecting your fertility as a couple.

The semen analysis tests for the following:

Sperm count. Having a low sperm count, called *oligospermia,* or an absence of sperm, *azospermia,* are the most obvious abnormal findings associated with infertility. Count refers to either the concentration (how densely populated they are) or total number of sperm in a specimen. The concentration is more predictive of a problem.

Sperm motility. This is a measure of how many sperm are moving and if they are moving forward and fast enough to penetrate an egg. This also calculates the percentage of sperm that are no longer viable. It's normal for some sperm to be dead or dying, but the majority should be alive and swimming at a good clip. If you have a normal sperm count, but low motility, you'll be diagnosed with *asthenospermia.* If there is very low motility, a follow-up test will be performed for sperm viability to see if more than 70 percent are dead, a condition called *necrospermia.*

Morphology. This judges the appearance of your sperm—their size, shape, and anatomy. It's normal for many sperm to appear imperfect, and often marginally abnormal sperm are categorized as abnormal. That's why the current guidelines (called the *Kruger strict criteria*) allow for up to 84 percent of the sperm to appear unusual in an otherwise "normal" specimen. But if 85 percent or more are abnormal, a condition called *teratospermia,* fertilization will be reduced.

Semen. The quantity and quality of the liquid portion of your specimen is also analyzed. A low volume suggests an incomplete collection (if a man misses the cup) or a short interval from your last ejaculation. If you continually have a very low volume, you may have *retrograde ejaculation.* During normal ejaculation, the opening of the bladder closes so that semen passing through the urethra doesn't enter the bladder. But if you have this condition, the bladder opening doesn't close properly, allowing sperm to enter the bladder instead of being ejaculated. To determine the quality of the sperm, there must be an adequate number of total sperm in the specimen, and the acid-base balance should

Ask Dr. Greene

Q Should my partner switch from briefs to boxers to improve his sperm count?

A You've probably heard that wearing loose boxers or using water-cooled athletic supporters can lower the temperature of your partner's testicles to improve sperm production. But the research shows that these efforts have no impact on the temperature of the testicles or sperm production. However, wearing tight jeans or Lycra cycling shorts can heat up the testicles, and have a negative effect on sperm production.

PASS ON POSTCOITAL TESTING

The postcoital test was once part of the standard workup for couples with infertility, but it has fallen out of favor among fertility specialists. However, many nonspecialists still perform this test, even though the ASRM has recommended against its use. For this test, typically performed shortly before ovulation, a woman has to go to the doctor's office between 2 and 12 hours after intercourse. The doctor collects a specimen in a test similar to a Pap smear, and the specimen is examined under a microscope for motile sperm. The test is very imprecise because the sperm may have already made it into the uterus by the time the specimen is taken, so a finding of no sperm doesn't mean anything. It's a waste of time and money. There's one exception: It's useful in couples who, for religious reasons, will not collect a specimen by masturbation or through the use of a condom.

lean more toward base. The base liquid provides a buffer for sperm against the mild acids in a woman's vagina. Semen also needs to coagulate to keep the sperm together for about 20 to 30 minutes after ejaculation, another protection against the acid pH of the vagina.

INSTRUCTIONS FOR SEMEN ANALYSIS

You can help improve the accuracy of your results. For the best results, follow these instructions.

- Your semen can vary considerably over time, so you should get two tests spaced at least a month apart to confirm an abnormal finding before you are diagnosed with a male factor. If your first finding is normal, you could start treatments based on your partner's factors, unless you'll feel more comfortable getting a confirmation of the normal result with a second test.
- Abstain from ejaculating two to five days prior to your test. With each day of abstinence (for up to a week) your sperm should increase by about 10 to 15 million. Your specimen should be analyzed by the lab within two hours of collection. If you're not collecting at the testing center, call ahead to be sure that they're expecting your specimen.

- The specimen should be collected either by masturbation or by using a special nonlatex condom during intercourse. Ordinary latex condoms impair sperm motility.
- The lab should provide you with a sterile, wide-mouthed specimen cup with a lid. You should also have a label to fill out with the date and time of collection and your identifying information.
- Keep the specimen around body temperature from the time of ejaculation until it is delivered to the laboratory by driving with the specimen between your legs or in a loose pocket. Keep notes of the time you dropped off your specimen.
- If the lab does not use computer-assisted semen analysis (CASA), ask for the name of the technician doing your evaluation. I recommend that you request the same technician during repeat examinations to maintain consistency from one examination to the next.
- If you do not collect the complete specimen, notify the lab or your health care provider. This is especially important since the first part of the ejaculate typically has the highest concentration of sperm.
- Do not use unapproved lubricants. There are some lubricants that won't harm sperm function, but most, including saliva, can create problems.
- Request a copy of your results for your records. Your results should include the following.

REFERENCE VALUES FOR STANDARD SEMEN ANALYSIS*

Parameters in **bold** are the most predictive factors.

Volume of ejaculate	1.5–5.0 ml
PH (acid-base balance)	>7.2 (neutral to base)
Concentration of sperm	>20 million/ml
Total number of sperm in specimen	>40 million/ejaculation
Percent motile	>50%
Forward progression**	>2 (scale 0–4)
Normal morphology**	>14%
Sperm agglutination**	<2 (scale 0–3)
Viscosity**	<h3 (scale 0–4)

*ASRM Practice Committee. Optimal Evaluation of the Infertile Male, Fertility Sterility 2006.
**Subjective assessment of the lab technician based upon established criteria.

ASSESSING YOUR SEMEN ANALYSIS

I have designated male factors 1 to 4 (from mild to severe) based on the results of a multicenter study published in 2001 by the National Cooperative Reproductive Medicine Network—a group of fertility centers whose goal is to increase the quality of research in the field of fertility. The researchers differentiated "fertility zones" for semen concentration, motility, and morphology characteristics. I have based the four fertility factor levels on these zones. Compare your semen analysis to the following table to identify your male factor.

DETERMINING MALE FACTOR

Select the number that correlates with each parameter for your semen analysis. Add the numbers together to create a total. Interpret your results with the scale listed below to learn more about your fertility status.

	0	1	2
Sperm concentration (million/ml)	>48.0	13.5–48.0	<13.5
Percent motile	>63	32–63	<32
Normal morphology	>12	9–12	<9

TOTAL SCORE: _____

Total your score. Here's the bottom line:

Score	Severity
0:	Male factor 1
1–2:	Male factor 2
3–4:	Male factor 3
5–6:	Male factor 4

Record your male factor in the chart on page 226 to help determine what level treatment you may need to consider. Then review the factors below to get a sense of how your factor will affect your chance of pregnancy.

Male Factor 1: Presumed Fertile

You have a normal semen analysis—very encouraging news, though it doesn't necessarily mean that your fertility issues rest entirely with your partner. Your treatments will be determined by your partner's fertility factors based on her testing. If those initial treatments aren't successful, then you may need to go through additional testing later. And even though your semen analysis is factor 1, other issues may impact your fertility and your treatment options.

Your biological clock. Recent studies have confirmed that men, too, have a "biological clock" ticking away as they age. Even with a reassuring semen analysis, you can have a reduced fertility rate and a higher risk of miscarriage, depending on your age. For men, there seems to be a noted change in fertility by age 40. This issue was rarely discussed in the past, since men can still father a pregnancy well into their 60s. But it came to light as more men over 40 began trying to conceive—and faced infertility. If you don't achieve results early in your treatment, your age may be a reason to move on to the next level of treatment sooner than a younger couple would.

Hormone balance. Continue to follow the Perfect Balance program to promote hormone balance. Subtle imbalances may arise that can contribute to your infertility. For instance, if your testosterone level drops, your libido may suffer; if your stress hormones become elevated, your sperm count may dip. Also avoid herbal supplements, some of which can interfere with hormone functioning.

Sexual function. An estimated 20 to 30 million men in the United States experience some form of sexual dysfunction, an obvious barrier to fertility. But up until the last decade, sexual dysfunction has been widely overlooked as a cause of infertility because of the sensitive nature of the topic and the stigma attached to it. Now it's spoken about more publicly, and the stigmatizing term "impotent" has been replaced by more descriptive medical terms like "erectile dysfunction," "low libido," "anorgasmia," and "premature ejaculation disorder." Each of these disorders can compromise your ability to conceive. Some forms may require fertility treatment to overcome, but in other cases, you may be able to treat the underlying sexual dysfunction and restore your fertility. Talk to your health care provider if you're experiencing a sexual dysfunction that has been interfering with successful intercourse.

BioMutagen exposure. Many effects of hormone disrupting agents and toxins don't impact sperm count, but they can influence pregnancy rates and the chance of a miscarriage. See Appendix B for a list of common BioMutagens to avoid. Additionally, avoid tobacco exposure, including secondhand smoke, since this is one of the most common toxins to healthy sperm function.

TOP 10 OCCUPATIONS ASSOCIATED WITH FERTILITY PROBLEMS

The first clues that certain BioMutagens interfered with male fertility came from studies looking at occupational exposure. Repeated exposure to minute quantities of a substance over time can wreak havoc on your reproductive system. Of the jobs that have been studied, these are most consistently associated with reproductive problems in men.

Occupation	Abnormal Semen Analysis	Decreased Pregnancy	Elevated Miscarriage
Conventional farming	+	+	+
Mechanics	+		+
Welding	+	+	
Plastics manufacturing	+		
Taxi/truck drivers	+		
Military service	+		
Printing/copying			+
Construction			+
Machinist			+
Tobacco processing			+

Male Factor 2: Mild

Many subtle changes to your hormones, your nutrition, or your metabolism can contribute to minor changes in your semen. Having male factor 2 does not mean that you absolutely need treatment to get pregnant. But I often recommend treatment, such as intrauterine insemination—when a man's purified sperm is instilled directly into his partner's uterus after she ovulates—as part of your combined treatment plan (see page 242 for more information). At this mild level, your best bet is to pursue this or other treatments, depending on your partner's female factors, rather than have any further testing for male factor infertility.

Case in Point

I met Sue, 28, and Steve, 32, after they had been trying to become pregnant for nearly six years. Sue had normal menstrual cycles and was ovulating monthly, but the doctor she was seeing put her on Clomid to produce additional eggs. After nearly a year of this treatment, she and Steve, completely frustrated, came to see me.

When I first met with them, I reviewed their medical tests and previous treatments. The only test that I wanted to repeat was Steve's semen analysis. I didn't trust the first test because CASA wasn't used. We repeated the test using CASA and found a very slight decrease in his sperm's motility, though everything else appeared normal. I categorized him as having male factor 2. I recommended combining Clomid to enhance ovulation with intrauterine insemination, making it easier for his slightly sluggish sperm to reach her egg. They became pregnant on their very first treatment cycle. Sue gave birth to a baby girl just after her due date. The story doesn't end here, though. When they were ready to have a second child, they tried on their own for 18 months before they came to see me again. Sue was nearly 35 and concerned that her age was causing the problem. I was not convinced, and rather than perform testing on her, I suggested they try the same exact treatment as before. On their second cycle, they conceived and had another healthy baby girl.

If you're male factor 2, continue to follow the Perfect Balance program, as these lifestyle factors may improve your sperm quality. Here are some other factors that can also impact your fertility.

Nutrition. In addition to following the nutritional advice in the program, you may benefit from getting more vitamin E, vitamin C, selenium, lycopene, L-carnitine, zinc, and folic acid—as these nutrients support healthy sperm production. I recommend the supplement ConceptionXR since it contains each of these ingredients.

BioMutagen exposure. Hormone-disrupting pollutants may play a role in your hormone balance. See Appendix B for a list of common BioMutagens to avoid.

Timing sex. Since you have a mild male factor, try to optimize your sperm count on the days that your partner is most fertile. Ask your

Fertility Fact

Lose Weight to Improve Fertility

Losing weight may be your greatest modifiable risk factor for infertility. Though testosterone naturally dips with age, a large study published in 2006 found that men who were 30 pounds overweight accelerated their testosterone loss by about 10 years. A drop in testosterone is associated with a drop in fertility and an increased risk of erectile dysfunction, fatigue, and low libido. Another study found that the more overweight men became, the greater their risk of male infertility. As you try to lose weight through the Perfect Balance program, your best measure of success is how many inches you lose around your waist, rather than how many pounds you drop on the scale.

partner when she is expecting to ovulate (she should be using an ovulation prediction kit), and try to have an ejaculation about five to seven days before that date, followed by abstinence until she ovulates or until your planned treatment.

Male Factor 3: Moderate

Your semen count is having a major impact on the fertility of you and your partner. Your partner should still do a complete evaluation before you begin considering treatment options to see if she has any female factors that are also contributing. You may be offered some additional tests as well, but some of these tests won't help determine pregnancy rates or treatment recommendations. Here are some areas to be aware of before you undergo any additional testing.

TESTOSTERONE DEFICIENCY: AN UNDERTREATED CONDITION

Testosterone naturally declines with age, but we're just beginning to realize the impact that this drop in testosterone has on male fertility. We now know that it can cause reduced sperm production, low libido, and erectile dysfunction. Low testosterone may also raise your risk of diabetes, heart disease, stroke, Alzheimer's disease, and Parkinson's disease. If you experience fatigue, weight gain, low libido, or erectile dysfunction, complete the "Androgen Deficiency Syndrome Questionnaire" on page 48 and then request a test for a blood level of "free and total testosterone" to see if you may benefit from taking Bioidentical testosterone.

EFFECT OF VARIOUS MEDICATIONS ON FERTILITY

Certain medications can affect a man's sperm count and function. Talk to your doctor if you're taking any of these.

Medication	Mechanism
Cimetidine Narcotic pain relievers Alkylating agents	Inhibit testosterone
Anabolic steroids	Inhibit FSH-LH release
Antiepilepsy drugs	Create estrogen-testosterone imbalance
Sulfasalazine Nitrofurantoin Thiazide diuretics	Impair sperm production
Calcium channel blockers Colchicine	Impair sperm function

Hormone balance. It's worth clarifying whether hormones have contributed to your moderate male factor since they are the most correctable aspect of your problem. I recommend an examination by a reproductive endocrinologist to determine if any hormone testing is indicated. This specialist would be most qualified to differentiate genetic problems or anatomic ones that may not be correctable.

BioMutagen exposure. This may play an even larger role in male factor 3 and male factor 4. Research shows that males who were exposed to hormone-disrupting agents while they were in the womb may have decreased fertility. For example, males that were exposed to substances like diethylstilbestrol (DES), a potent synthetic estrogen given to pregnant women from 1940 through the 1960s, have about a 30 percent increased risk of infertility. The good news is that they still respond very well to treatment. If you have access to information about possible toxins you were exposed to as a child or during your own fetal development, discuss them with your doctor.

Anatomic abnormalities. One factor that may be contributing to male factor 3 is the presence of a *varicocele,* an enlargement of the scrotal veins that results in blood pressure or temperature changes

FERTILITY AFTER CANCER TREATMENT

Over 800,000 reproductive age women and men in the United States have cancer. By 2010, it's estimated that 1 of every 250 adults will be a survivor of childhood cancers. The National Cancer Institute recommends that when considering cancer treatments, reproductive issues should be discussed with patients. Many cancer treatments entail chemotherapy or radiation therapy or both. High doses of the chemotherapies classified as alkylating agents are the most damaging to sperm production. But with these agents, as with other chemotherapy drugs, studies suggest that when sperm function returns, there is a low risk of genetic damage. Additionally, being pretreated with hormones that suppress sperm production can further reduce the risk of fertility problems (this, in effect, rests the cells so they are less susceptible to the chemotherapy). Radiation therapy, either to the gonads or to the head in children that haven't gone through puberty, tends to have a more damaging effect on reproductive function. Newer research suggests that damage can be minimized by narrowing the radiation field and possibly through the use of hormone suppression as well.

If you've been treated for cancer, obtain a copy of your records to determine what your cancer treatment entailed. This will provide the greatest prognostic information for you and your partner. If you've recently been diagnosed with cancer, I recommend that you review the People Living with Cancer website (www.plwc.org) of the American Society of Clinical Oncology for information on fertility preservation. By planning ahead, you can reduce your risk of having fertility issues later.

within the testicles. This common abnormality occurs in about 15 percent of fertile men, but in about 45 percent of men with infertility. A varicocele is often palpable—it feels like several soft noodle-like structures in the scrotum. There is considerable debate about the effectiveness of correcting a varicocele since other nonsurgical treatments may be more effective at helping you and your partner become pregnant. Consider consulting with a urologist familiar with this procedure, as well as a reproductive endocrinologist, in order to get both views on the usefulness of this surgery.

General health. A number of health conditions (or their treatments) can compromise fertility. If you have a known health problem or unexplained symptoms, get a complete physical examination if you haven't already. If you do have a disorder, tell your doctor that you and your partner are trying to get pregnant because it may impact the medication or dose you're given. Some common health ailments can affect your fertility in the following ways.

- A *high fever* can markedly diminish sperm quality for three to six months after you recover.
- *Prostatitis, sexually transmitted diseases like gonorrhea, or any infection* that increases the number of white blood cells present in the ejaculated specimen can markedly diminish the ability of sperm to fertilize an egg. These infections can be treated, so see a urologist if you're having trouble urinating, have a history of any of these infections, or if your semen analysis detected white blood cells.
- *Diabetes* needs to be well controlled to reduce your risk of developing erectile dysfunction or vascular problems that can diminish sperm production. If your blood sugar has been poorly controlled, it's time to get serious about managing your condition.
- *High blood pressure, high cholesterol, or known vascular disease* can impact the blood vessels that supply the testicles and interfere with sperm production. Talk to your doctor about steps you can take to manage these conditions.
- *Epilepsy or other brain disorders* can often be associated with a reduction in sperm production. Usually, the treatment contributes to the problem. Talk to your doctor about whether it may be appropriate to lower your dose of medication or switch to another as you try to conceive.

Immunologic reactions. Antisperm antibodies—small proteins that can attach to sperm and dramatically impair their ability to fertilize an egg—may contribute to infertility for up to 20 percent of men with moderate to severe infertility, compared to about 2 percent of men that don't have infertility. Though suppressing antibodies may be offered to you as a treatment, the best approach is to select the appropriate assisted reproductive technology (ART) in order to circumvent this issue.

Male Factor 4: Severe

You likely have an anatomical problem that is preventing your sperm from moving from the testicles to the epididymis to be ejaculated. In some cases, you may have inherited a genetic abnormality, preventing sperm from functioning. You will need ART in order to conceive, and even some of these treatments may not work for you. Instead, you may choose to use a sperm donor, which would mean that no additional evaluation is necessary. If you and your partner are open to considering this option, you should do so before moving forward with additional testing or treatment in order to save considerable time and money. If you do choose to investigate treatment options that would make it possible to use your sperm, here are some points you should consider.

Anatomic abnormalities. The major anatomic problems are:

- *Previous vasectomy.* A vasectomy involves cutting the two *vas deferens* tubes so that sperm cannot get into the semen. Some men ultimately regret having a vasectomy because they later decide they want to have more children. Vasectomy reversal comes with a 20 percent risk of not restoring sperm to the ejaculate. You may also confront new issues; for instance, some men begin to form antibodies to their sperm, while others experience a reduction in sperm production over time from the effects of the surgery. In the past, a reversal was the only option, but today couples generally have a much higher success rate at a lower cost by turning to ART instead (see chapter 14). Procedures involve obtaining sperm surgically and using them to directly fertilize an egg. Before you consider having reversal surgery, consult with both a urologist and a reproductive endocrinologist to get perspectives on surgery versus ART.

- *Congenital bilateral absence of vas deferens (CBAVD).* About 1 to 2 percent of men with severe male factor infertility were born without the vas deferens. Your doctor can detect CBAVD through a careful examination. This birth defect is often associated with being a carrier of the cystic fibrosis gene, so if you have it, your partner should be tested for the cystic fibrosis gene as well; if you are both carriers, the risk of your offspring having cystic fibrosis is at least 50 percent. With today's advanced genetic testing methods, you can undergo IVF and have the embryos tested prior to selection and transfer.

- *Retrograde ejaculation.* This fairly common disorder, in which the sperm enters the bladder (see page 143), is associated with

Case in Point

After having three children with his first wife, Ethan had a vasectomy. But a few years later, he and his wife divorced, and he later met Nicole, who was widowed at 35 and had two children of her own. A year into their marriage, Ethan went to his urologist to discuss a vasectomy reversal. Despite the 20 percent risk of failure, Ethan chose the reversal surgery. The procedure went well and the doctor confirmed sperm were present at the time of surgery. But tests at three and six months after the surgery found sperm were no longer present.

With the best of intentions, Ethan's urologist offered to do a repeat reversal. They were counseled that repeat surgeries had an even higher failure rate, but that they were often successful. (The fact is, no good statistics exist for repeat procedures because of the many variables involved, such as the age of the male, the amount of time since the original procedure, and the techniques used.) But not knowing this, they decided to go for it—but again the surgery failed. About a year passed before they decided to pursue ART and contacted my office.

At the time I met Ethan and Nicole, he was 45 and she had just turned 39. I suggested that we proceed directly to an advanced technique that involved retrieval of his sperm through a mild surgical procedure called percutaneous epididymal sperm aspiration (PESA) in combination with an IVF cycle. We could then place a single sperm directly inside each egg we retrieved from Nicole. The procedures yielded eight embryos, and two were transferred to Nicole's womb. One embryo implanted, and Nicole gave birth to a healthy girl.

diabetes, spinal cord injury, or previous pelvic surgery in men. It can be diagnosed by performing a urine analysis after ejaculation to determine if sperm are present. If so, there are many treatment options available. The most common is to empty your bladder prior to ejaculating, and then provide a urine specimen, from which sperm can be isolated.

- *Acquired ejaculatory duct obstruction.* Sperm are transported via the vas deferens to the ejaculatory ducts. A blockage would keep sperm from passing through the duct during ejaculation. This is typically due to certain pelvic infections, severe injury to the gonads, or previous surgery. You wouldn't know if you had a blockage because you would ejaculate semen. To determine if you have a blockage, you may have your semen tested for fructose, a natural sugar that's added to the ejaculate during sperm production. Though sperm can be blocked from getting through, traces of fructose will if you are ejaculating semen. A positive fructose test with no sperm present indicates a blockage preventing sperm from leaving your testicles. This problem may be correctable by surgery or through the use of advanced reproductive procedures.

Your genes. A new breed of testing for minor genetic abnormalities, called *sperm DNA integrity testing,* has recently become available. Research has found that when tested, 15 percent of fertile men test positive for minor DNA abnormalities, whereas 30 percent of infertile men test positive. Still, these tests are *not* recommended by ASRM because the results have not been shown to affect pregnancy prognosis or to guide treatment options. If your physician recommends this test, inquire what the benefit would be and if the results would change his course of treatment.

General health. Your health may be compounding your problem. Review general health recommendations for male factor 3 and then talk to your doctor.

Immunologic reactions. As I described for men with male factor 3, in up to 20 percent of men with severe infertility, antibodies may be contributing to the problem. If you have male factor 4, this is not likely to be the only cause of your fertility problems. Current recommendations are to select the appropriate ART that circumvents the antibody issue.

BEFORE YOU PROCEED WITH TREATMENT

I don't recommend that you move forward with treatment until both of you complete your examinations. In the following chapters, I will provide similar guidelines regarding the factors that may affect female fertility. I have divided these into separate chapters for ovarian factor, tubal factor, uterine factor, and other factors. Only when you have all of that information will you be fully prepared to make informed decisions about which treatment option will be most appropriate for both of you.

9 Ovarian Factor

The first place to look when you're having fertility issues is your ovaries, home to hundreds of thousands of your microscopic eggs, each containing your genetic contribution to your future child. Your two ovaries, each the size of a large olive, are great multitaskers. Not only do they nest and nourish your eggs, but acting as endocrine glands, they coordinate all of the early hormonal changes necessary to support implantation and fetal development. Given these critical roles, it's no surprise that an estimated 40 percent of female infertility is related to the inability of ovaries to produce and nurture a fertilizable egg. The incidence of ovarian dysfunction is rising as more couples choose to have children later in life—the older ovary and the older eggs it nests are prone to more problems. The good news is that in today's fertility clinics, there are a growing number of treatments available to overcome ovarian infertility. Before initiating treatment, it is important to understand how well your ovaries function to produce healthy eggs, promote ovulation, and maintain hormone balance.

> ## Did you know ?
>
> The time it takes an egg to go from dormancy to ovulation is about equal to the length of a full-term pregnancy.

OVULATION

You are born with about 2 million eggs, but you will only ovulate about 400 eggs in your lifetime. Each egg is dormant, nestled within its own cocoon of fluid and covered by a thin outer shell. It can survive approximately four decades after puberty. In this state, the cocooned eggs are called *primordial follicles,* but in any given month, a follicle may become activated and go through a series of events leading to either ovulation or death. As you'll see in the time line that follows, numerous hormonal signals are exchanged within the ovary and between the ovary and the brain.

COUNTDOWN TO OVULATION

Refer back to this countdown as you read this chapter and consider your ovarian factors.

290 Days Before Conception
* Dormant primordial follicles activate their DNA, kicking off the 290-day process of maturation.

3 Months Before Conception
* Hormones signal about a dozen of these activated eggs to advance to the next stage of maturation. The group of eggs is called a *cohort.*
* Now referred to as *primary follicles,* they begin to expand with fluids chock-full of hormones and nutrients to support their growth. The egg appears as if it is suspended in a small puddle of fluid.
* A layer of hormone-producing specialized cells called *granulosa* cells forms the outer wall of each follicle to encase the egg.

2 Months Before Conception
* The layer of granulosa cells begins to thicken to nine layers deep; these cells produce estradiol and more fluid.
* *Thecal cells,* another type of specialized cell in the ovary, encourage small blood vessels to grow to support the development of the follicles, now considered *secondary follicles.*

2 to 3 Weeks Before Conception
* Growing follicles, called *antral follicles,* can now be seen on an ultrasound.
* Only five to seven follicles from the original cohort typically remain.

Menstrual Day 1: Your Period
* The day your menstrual cycle begins is the first day of your period. Your period signals the beginning of the 14-day *follicular phase,* during which the antral follicles begin to compete with one another for dominance.

- Your levels of estradiol and progesterone have hit their nadir. Over the next two weeks, these hormones will rise again, preparing for ovulation and pregnancy.
- Your brain sends LH pulses to specialized thecal cells, instructing them to convert cholesterol into testosterone. Granulosa cells in turn convert the testosterone into estradiol, creating a gradual rise in estradiol that will eventually trigger ovulation.

Menstrual Day 2 to 4

- A few of the antral follicles are now recruited (in response to the hormonal signals) to complete this journey.
- Increasing levels of FSH help the eggs mature and begin to produce estradiol.
- Follicles produce hormones like *inhibin B* and *Müllerian inhibiting hormone*, which suppress the other follicles in their battle for dominance.

Menstrual Day 5 to 7

- As antral follicles grow, they send more and more estradiol to your hypothalamus.
- FSH signals the follicles to produce fluid more rapidly, helping follicles grow.

Menstrual Day 8

- By now, one follicle has reached the size of a pea (about 1 centimeter, or cm) and can produce enough hormones to suppress the other remaining follicles. It is clearly recognized on an ultrasound as the dominant follicle.
- Within the fluid of the dominant follicle, the egg is bathed in FSH, estradiol, and progesterone. The fluid of the smaller, regressing follicles has low levels of estradiol and high levels of prolactin and testosterone, hormones that play a role in their atrophy.

Menstrual Day 12: Ovulation

- The dominant follicle is now the size of a nickel (about 2 cm), though the egg within the fluid is only about the size of the period at the end of this sentence.
- Once levels of estradiol reach at least 200 pg/ml (picogram/milliliter) for more than 50 hours, your pituitary sends a surge of LH, preparing the dominant follicle for ovulation. This signal typically occurs in the early predawn hours.
- A cascade of chemical changes erodes the follicle wall to liberate the egg from its watery lair. Ovulation occurs 34 to 36 hours after the spike in LH.
- The fertile egg then enters the fallopian tube, where it must be penetrated by the awaiting sperm within about a day, or the window of opportunity will close and the egg will atrophy.

OVARIAN FACTORS

To assess your ovarian factor and its severity, you need to establish whether you have any of the following problems. Once you review these sections and determine which symptoms, if any, you have, you

THE HORMONE PLAYERS

◆ **Estradiol,** the most potent form of estrogen, helps the brain monitor egg development, and signals the brain to trigger ovulation.

◆ **Follicle-stimulating hormone (FSH)** is released by the brain's pituitary, primarily in the first 10 days and last few days of a woman's cycle. FSH signals the ovaries to prepare eggs for ovulation.

◆ **Luteinizing hormone (LH)** is released by the pituitary in low levels throughout the month, but in a surge just before ovulation, signaling a developing follicle to release the egg. LH also promotes the production of estradiol by the ovary.

◆ **Gonadotropin-releasing hormone (GnRH),** released by the hypothalamus, triggers the pituitary to release FSH and LH.

◆ **Progesterone** rises for seven to eight days after ovulation and prepares the lining of the uterus for implantation and pregnancy. Progesterone is essential for maintaining a pregnancy.

◆ **Prolactin,** released by the pituitary, normally rises during pregnancy and breast-feeding, signaling the ovaries that conditions are not right for another pregnancy at the moment. Sustained prolactin release, which also occurs under stress, inhibits ovulation by suppressing the release of FSH and GnRH.

will be able to plug that information into the "Ovarian Factor Questionnaire" on page 167 to determine if you have an ovarian factor and its level of severity.

1. Do You Have a Regular Menstrual Cycle?

Your menstrual cycle offers one of the clearest insights into your fertility. If you get your period regularly, every 28 days or so, there is a 95 percent chance that you're ovulating. Having irregular menstrual cycles that vary in length, or infrequent menstrual cycles are fairly common problems in women with infertility. *Amenorrhea,* having no menstrual cycle for at least three months, is a less-common but more-serious indicator of hormone imbalance and infertility. Use the fertility calendar in Appendix A to track your menstrual cycles, the day your period starts, and the day it ends. Record the frequency of your cycles in the questionnaire on page 167.

2. Are You Ovulating?

Ovulation requires near-perfect hormonal balance. This balance is characterized by low stress hormones, adequate levels of thyroid hormones, an absence of insulin resistance, and low levels of prolactin, a hormone often released under stress. For many women, this state of equilibrium comes naturally, resulting in regularly spaced menstrual cycles and monthly ovulation. For some, though, hormonal stability is more precarious, leading to irregular menstrual cycles and inconsistent ovulatory patterns. Still others have profound hormonal imbalances, causing an environment in which an egg cannot develop properly, and resulting in only the rare release of a mature egg. My program will help you establish the best hormonal balance you can. But for about one in nine couples with infertility, this still won't be enough to overcome more profound ovulatory disturbances. You can monitor your ovulation by using the Clearblue Easy Fertility Monitor or the OV-Watch, for three to four months (see page 119 for a complete description). If you're not menstruating, you're probably not ovulating either. Record your ovulation frequency in the questionnaire on page 167.

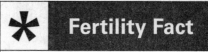

Fertility Fact

Low Iron, Low Fertility

In 2006, the results of the large-scale Nurses' Health Study II clearly demonstrated the importance of iron supplementation on a woman's fertility. In 1989, this study enrolled nearly 20,000 married women of reproductive age with no history of infertility. The researchers found that women taking a supplement with high iron content had about a 70 percent lower risk of ovulatory infertility. Aside from carrying oxygen in the blood, iron is also used by granulosa cells and eggs to make key proteins that help the egg mature. Since iron deficiency was not tested in this study, it's difficult to say if all women share the benefit of an iron supplement or only women with iron deficiency (anemia). However, one in five reproductive-age women in the United States have low iron stores. Until more is known, you might benefit from either taking a supplement or requesting a blood test for iron (serum ferritin). If your ferritin is less than 12 ng/ml, then you'll need a supplement. I recommend Repliva, as it is easily absorbed and well tolerated.

RULE OUT LUTEAL INSUFFICIENCY

The luteal phase, between ovulation and your first day of menstruation, is typically 14 days long. If you find that fewer than 14 days pass from the time of ovulation to the onset of your period, you may have a problem that can interfere with implantation of a pregnancy (refer to chapter 11). Keep a record of your ovulation date and the date that your period begins in your fertility calendar.

3. Do You Have Polycystic Ovarian Syndrome?

The most common cause of missed periods is *polycystic ovarian syndrome*, or *PCOS*, affecting more than 6 million women in the United States. One of the biggest problems in the field of fertility today is that many doctors are not recognizing PCOS in their patients. Although doctors tend to be aware of the most common visible symptoms—being overweight, and having excess hair and acne—many don't realize that thin patients and others without these classic symptoms can have PCOS as well. I encourage you to take an active role in assessing whether you have this condition to avoid going undiagnosed or mistakenly receiving the diagnosis of "unexplained infertility."

If you have missed periods or if there is any evidence that you're not ovulating, your first step should be to request an evaluation for PCOS. This syndrome is characterized by high testosterone production (causing the acne and the hair growth), irregular ovulation, and multiple small cysts on the ovary, called *polycystic ovaries* (PCO). These small cysts are partially developed follicles that have stopped maturing because of the inhibitory effects of the high testosterone levels. A woman needs to have two of these three factors to meet the criteria for the diagnosis.

Here's how you can evaluate whether you have any of the three factors.

Excess testosterone, or hyperandrogenism. Symptoms that are highly suggestive of elevated testosterone are acne and excess hair growth. If you have either of these symptoms, then you do not need a blood test to confirm high testosterone, since they indicate that you're sensitive to the amount of testosterone present in your blood regardless of the amount. If you don't have these symptoms, request the blood test for total and free testosterone. High insulin levels, cre-

Case in Point

At 22, Rachael was diagnosed with PCOS. She had irregular, infrequent menstrual cycles and excessive hair growth and acne. Her doctor placed her on a birth control pill to help regulate the menstrual cycles and even help her acne, but no effort was made to treat the underlying insulin resistance, which is at the root of PCOS. At 25, she married Alex, and soon went off her birth control pill to try to become pregnant. After several missed menstrual cycles and negative pregnancy tests, she went back to her doctor, who told her that she was having trouble because she was overweight—another symptom of PCOS—and placed her on a synthetic progestin, called Provera, to induce a menstrual cycle (he didn't tell her that Provera worsens insulin resistance). She later told me that each time she had to take Provera, she would gain even more weight. Three years had passed with continued weight gain and the disappointment of no pregnancy when Rachael made an appointment at my office.

I confirmed her diagnosis of PCOS and ordered blood tests to see what underlying imbalances were causing the disorder. These tests showed that she had significant insulin resistance and mild hypothyroidism. The cumulative effect had increased her testosterone level, causing the excess hair growth and acne, and reducing her chance of ovulation. We began treatment by inducing a menstrual cycle with the BioIdentical progesterone called Prometrium, which doesn't worsen insulin resistance. I also started her on an insulin-sensitizing BioModifier, metformin, to improve her insulin resistance, and the BioIdentical thyroid replacement hormone called Thyrolar.

Rachael met with my nutritionist to learn how to improve her dietary choices to lose weight. She also began taking daily walks. In three months, she lost 12 pounds and had a menstrual cycle. But after three more months, she only had one more menstrual cycle, and wanted to begin fertility treatment. We tried to induce ovulation with Clomid, but when her ovaries didn't respond, we switched to another ovulation induction drug, the low-dose BioIdentical FSH called Follistim. On the third cycle, Rachael conceived. She continued taking metformin throughout the pregnancy and delivered a healthy boy.

ated by insulin resistance, are the most common reason women have high testosterone.

Anovulation. This is defined as having infrequent menstrual cycles, irregular cycles, or menstruating without ovulating. Use an at-home ovulation prediction kit for three to four months to monitor your ovulation.

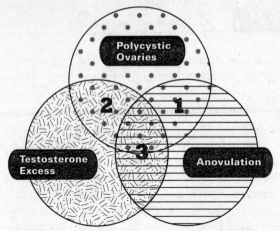

(Modified from the Rotterdam Criteria for Diagnosing PCOS.)

PCOS is a symptom-based diagnosis. The symptoms often overlap into three zones. The zone you fall into reflects the severity of your symptoms. Use this diagram to determine your zone; then refer to the key below to understand the implications of your symptoms. If you have one of these symptoms, but are uncertain about whether you have any other symptoms, request an evaluation for the other two factors. If you fall into any zone, complete the "Insulin Resistance Risk Questionnaire" on page 41 to estimate your level of insulin resistance. Record your zone in the "Ovarian Factor Questionnaire" on page 167.

    Zone 1: Mild PCOS. If you don't ovulate consistently, and you have polycystic ovaries, you may have mild PCOS. You are at the highest risk of not being diagnosed because your symptoms are so subtle. You probably have mild insulin resistance as the primary trigger of your hormone imbalance. It may become more advanced with time, so it's important to follow the Perfect Balance program; a poor diet and unhealthy lifestyle can easily nudge you into full-blown PCOS.

    Zone 2: Moderate PCOS. You ovulate consistently, but have polycystic ovaries and problems due to excess testosterone. Your insulin resistance is definitely a factor contributing to your symptoms and your infertility.

    Zone 3: Severe PCOS. You do not ovulate, you have excess testosterone, and you may or may not have polycystic ovaries. This is contributing to your infertility.

Polycystic ovaries. Cysts can only be detected with an ultrasound or other imaging test, but testing is not necessary to confirm PCOS, unless your diagnosis cannot be determined by other factors. If you're having an ultrasound for another reason, your health care provider should examine your ovaries. If your ovaries are larger than 10 cc (cubic centimeters) or have more than 12 antral follicles early in your cycle, you have polycystic ovaries.

4. Do You Have a Healthy Ovarian Reserve (Is Your Biological Clock Ticking)?

Your ovarian reserve, popularly referred to as your biological clock, is a rough estimate of how rapidly your fertility is declining. Specifi-

THE HORMONE THAT CAUSES ANOVULATION

New research has found that the underlying cause of anovulation may be anti-Müllerian hormone (AMH), a hormone produced by granulosa cells in the follicles from very early in follicle development until the antral stage. But AMH is thought to stop the development of neighboring follicles. Recall that cysts are follicles that have stopped developing; however, they do continue to secrete AMH, creating high levels of the hormone. Testing for AMH is not typically done unless you're getting advanced testing for ovarian reserve (the number of eggs you have remaining). If you have this test, and your AMH is high, it's a sign of PCOS. Women with mild PCOS have AMH levels about 3 to 4 times above average and those with severe PCOS have levels that are 75 times higher.

cally, ovarian reserve describes how many high-quality eggs remain in your ovaries. This is essential in determining your ovarian factor. During your early and mid-reproductive years, the highest-quality eggs respond most readily to the hormonal triggers of ovulation. With age, the number of eggs—and the number of high-quality eggs—declines. On average, it's estimated that a woman in her late 30s has about 25,000 eggs left; but in her 40s, the numbers drop dramatically, so that as she approaches age 51, the typical age of menopause, she only has about 1,000 left. The rate of decline can vary depending on the following factors—some that are unalterable and others that you can control:

Genes account for 50 to 70 percent of your predicted fertile years. It's believed that genes located primarily on the X chromosome establish the rate at which your eggs must either ovulate or self-destruct. Your best estimate of your biological clock is the age that your mother and maternal grandmother entered menopause—but only if their menopause wasn't hastened by surgery or another unnatural cause.

Age determines the number of eggs you have remaining, but it also affects how your brain recruits follicles. It is believed that about 13 years prior to menopause, women experience a marked rise in follicle recruitment. Studies suggest that at this turning point, FSH increases, activating more eggs each month—this also happens to be the cause for the natural rise in the rate of multiple births as women age.

Medical history impacts your ovaries and your fertility. If you're a type 1 or type 2 diabetic and have had poorly controlled blood sugar, it will reduce your number of fertile years because of insulin's negative impact on the ovary. If you've had poorly controlled epilepsy, the number of seizures that you had will proportionately bring on menopause earlier. Even a history of autoimmune disease, cancer, or pelvic surgery can cause early egg loss. Talk with your fertility specialist about any health condition you've had. Be sure to discuss any medications you've taken, as some can impact your ovaries as well.

BioMutagen exposure has a lasting effect on your ovarian reserve. Women that have smoked tend to enter menopause at least two years earlier than women that never used tobacco. Numerous studies have also found that exposure to pesticides and other hormone disrupting agents can impact your ovaries. Review Appendix B for a list of BioMutagens that can affect your fertility.

Egg quality worsens with age. Studies show that the outer membrane of the follicle becomes thicker and tougher over time, making it harder for sperm to penetrate. The eggs you ovulated 10 years ago would have been more easily fertilized than the ones you have today. Fertility treatments designed to overcome this functional change are typically offered to women over 35 who undergo IVF.

OVARIAN RESERVE TESTING

To help estimate your ovarian reserve, request a blood test of your serum estradiol and FSH levels. This inexpensive test is used to predict your chance of conception, but not whether you definitely can or can't conceive. Additional testing may be needed, depending on how you score on your ovarian factor questionnaire. Your blood test may need to be timed to day 3 of your menstrual cycle. The day your menstrual cycle begins is considered menstrual day 1 (if bleeding occurs after 8 p.m., count the next day as your first day). Request your lab slip ahead of time to be prepared. Don't forget to request a copy of your results.

FSH Results
- <9.0 IU/l: Your ovaries are still very sensitive to FSH and therefore able to respond to subtle messages from your brain to promote follicle maturation.

- 9.1 to 12.0 IU/l: Your ovaries are becoming less sensitive, requiring your brain to send a stronger signal to promote follicle growth.
- 12.1 to 16 IU/l: Your chance of pregnancy is low, and you should get further testing.
- >16.0 IU/l: Your chance of conception is low even with treatment.

Estradiol Results

- <50 pg/ml: Your ovaries are returning to the baseline starting point as you begin your menstrual cycle. They are fertile and responding appropriately.
- 50 to 80 pg/ml: You have early signs of reduced ovarian responsiveness.
- 81 to 100 pg/ml: Your follicles are not maturing appropriately. This also makes the FSH score less accurate for interpretation.
- >100 pg/ml: You may have an ovarian cyst or other source of estradiol.

OVARIAN FACTOR QUESTIONNAIRE

Use this questionnaire to help you understand where you are on the continuum of ovarian health. Your ovarian factor is based on the information you have gathered on your menstrual cycles, ovulation, the presence of PCOS and its severity, your ovarian reserve scores, and your age. Circle the answer that most accurately describes you.

	1	2	3	4
My menstrual cycles occur . . .	monthly	irregularly	infrequently	rarely
I ovulate . . .	monthly	most months	occasionally	never
Do you have PCOS?	No	Mild	Moderate	Severe
My FSH level is _____ IU/l	<9.0	9.1–12	12.1–16	>16.0
My serum estradiol level is _____ pg/ml	<50	51–80	81–100	>100
My current age is . . .	<35	35–37	38–42	>42

Total your score. Here's the bottom line:

Score	Severity
6–7:	Ovarian factor 1
8–10:	Ovarian factor 2
11–15:	Ovarian factor 3
16 or higher:	Ovarian factor 4

Record your ovarian factor in the chart on page 226 to help determine what treatment level you might want to consider.

Ovarian Factor 1: Presumed Fertile

This is very reassuring, and means that your ovarian health should not factor into your fertility options. It's not a guarantee that you don't have a subtle disturbance of ovulation or hormone production, but it's close to one. You should continue to take steps to minimize your BioMutagen exposure in order to protect your ovaries.

Ovarian Factor 2: Mild

Your ovaries should be factored into treatment as they are mildly impacting your ability to conceive. It may become more of an issue if you decide to have future pregnancies. What has a mild impact now could have a moderate impact in several years as you—and your ovaries—age. Though it isn't necessary now, you should consider advanced testing for ovarian reserve (see "Advanced Testing for Diminished Ovarian Reserve," page 169) for future pregnancies.

CANCER PATIENTS CAN PRESERVE THEIR FERTILITY

A cancer diagnosis in a young woman used to mean that she wouldn't be able to have children. With today's technology, cancer patients can take steps to preserve their fertility before treatment. Chemotherapy and radiation can speed the loss of follicles, putting women into *premature ovarian failure (POF)*, defined as entering menopause before age 40. POF is diagnosed by confirming elevated FSH and LH levels in a woman who stops menstruating for at least three months. Although this typically signifies the end of a woman's fertility, pregnancies do occur, even in the absence of treatment, in about 6 percent of women with this condition. If you have POF, see a board-certified reproductive endocrinologist to have a thorough evaluation and discuss treatments. If you've been diagnosed with cancer and haven't yet gone through treatment, see a fertility specialist before you begin treatment to discuss your options to prolong your fertility. These include freezing unfertilized eggs or slivers of ovarian tissue, banking embryos, relocating ovaries outside potential fields of radiation, or suppressing the ovaries with BioAntagonists or BioLimited hormones prior to exposing them to chemotherapy.

ADVANCED TESTING FOR DIMINISHED OVARIAN RESERVE

If you have ovarian factor 3 or 4, I recommend you talk to your specialist about which of the following tests you should complete. No single test is best for all women. I prefer a combination of the ultrasound and the AMH test. Together, they provide the best information for recommending treatment options at the lowest cost.

◆ **Ultrasound** (sometimes referred to as sonography) is a noninvasive way to examine your ovaries and take measurements that may predict your response to treatment. It should be performed on day 3 to 5 of your menstrual cycle. If your ovaries are smaller than 3 cc or have less than five antral follicles, you have a reduced ovarian reserve. Further testing may be warranted. If you're considering an ultrasound, first see if you'll also need one to examine your fallopian tubes or uterus (see chapters 10 and 11). As I mentioned, if you do one ultrasound to assess the three factors, it's a huge money saver.

◆ **Anti-Müllerian inhibiting hormone (AMH)** is a hormone produced by granulosa cells in follicles. This hormone inhibits adjacent follicles from maturing and remains at a stable level throughout the cycle. Very low levels suggest a reduced ovarian reserve (high levels suggest PCOS). Since your values remain stable throughout your cycle, this test can be combined with any other blood test you need rather than timed to a specific day of your menstrual cycle.

◆ **Inhibin B** is a hormone produced by the granulosa cells of small antral follicles. High inhibin-B early in the cycle (it's typically measured on menstrual day 5) means more antral follicles are present, which is good. Since aging of the ovaries is associated with a reduction in the number of antral follicles starting out a cycle, a low inhibin-B level predicts low ovarian reserve and a reduced response to fertility treatment.

◆ **Provocative testing** refers to the practice of administering a hormone and then measuring how your ovaries respond to it. These tests are typically named for the hormone used and have acronyms like CCCT, EFFORT, and GAST. I believe that for many couples, it's better to undergo a cycle of ovulation induction instead of these tests, since the treatment can provide the same information as the tests, and may even result in a pregnancy. These tests employ various combinations of blood tests and ultrasound examinations, and fertility specialists continue to debate which combination is the best. If your health care provider suggests provocative testing, ask him what guided his recommendation to be sure that your money is being well spent on the most appropriate test for you.

Ovarian Factor 3: Moderate

The quality of your follicles is a significant factor in your ability to conceive. In order to get the most appropriate treatment for your needs, you should see a board-certified reproductive endocrinologist and undergo more advanced testing for ovarian reserve (see "Advanced Testing for Diminished Ovarian Reserve" on page 169). If your goal is to have more than one pregnancy, you may want to have your eggs or embryos frozen and stored to improve your options later. These options are discussed further in chapter 14.

Ovarian Factor 4: Severe

If you have severe ovarian factor, your ovaries are a major obstacle to becoming pregnant. Additional testing will clarify whether you should even consider treatments, or whether you should pursue other alternatives like the use of donated eggs or embryos or adoption. Only a board-certified reproductive endocrinologist is qualified to thoroughly evaluate and discuss your treatment options. By seeking out all of the necessary information, and reviewing your options before your office visit, you can direct your first meeting based upon the emerging treatment options that are most appealing to you and your partner.

◆　◆　◆

Your ovaries play a central role in providing healthy DNA to your child as well as the hormones that are necessary to support the pregnancy. You can optimize their health and functioning by taking a prenatal vitamin and creating a healthy hormonal environment for them. In Part Four, "Your Fertility Plan: Making it Happen," I describe treatments that can help you overcome what used to be insurmountable fertility problems. But first, before you talk with a fertility specialist, review the chapters on all other factors to determine if you have any other obstacles to getting pregnant.

10 Tubal Factor

Your fallopian tubes are intricate, pencil-thin, life-preserving passageways between your ovaries and your uterus. Their lush environment is like a health spa, nourishing sperm as they await your ovulated egg, and extending their lives by as many as five days. It is in one of your two fallopian tubes that fertilization takes place, and where the developing embryo is then incubated for the first four or five days of life. The fallopian tube, about the length of a crayon, begins thin and narrow at your uterus, and gradually flares out like a trumpet, providing a wide opening to catch the egg as it's released from your ovary (the medical name for the

THE HORMONE PLAYERS

- ◆ **Progesterone.** During the first few days after fertilization, the early embryo has progesterone-secreting cells attached. The tiny amount of progesterone they produce may serve to slow the embryo's pace through the tube, allowing time for the endometrium to get primed and ready for implantation.

- ◆ **Estradiol.** After an initial dip following ovulation, estradiol remains elevated. It dilates blood vessels, promoting blood flow to the uterus, fallopian tubes, and ovaries.

tube is *salpinx,* Greek for "trumpeter"). But the dense anatomy of the fallopian tubes that makes them such a rich and safe haven for sperm, egg, and embryo also makes them more vulnerable to infection, injury, and obstruction.

A TALE OF TWO JOURNEYS

Sperm to Egg

Before sperm reach a fallopian tube, they need to traverse the uterus. It is believed that waves of contractions within the uterus propel sperm toward the fallopian tube that is receiving the released egg. Once sperm pass through the tube's portal, their progress is slowed by the dense, hairlike structures called *cilia* that line the length of the tube and provide nutrients and fluid for sperm and embryos. During this leg of the journey, a sperm has to complete two final steps of maturation before it meets an egg: *capacitation* and *hyperactivation.*

During capacitation, the sperm sheds proteins and cholesterol from its outer membrane, allowing it to bind to and penetrate an egg. In hyperactivation, the sperm's tail beats faster, increasing its speed and agility so it can sprint toward the awaiting egg and generate enough force to penetrate the egg's membrane. Sperm approach the end of the fallopian tube in waves in order to ensure a fresh band of active sperm is present whenever the egg appears.

Egg to Embryo to Womb

The trumpeted or *distal* end of the fallopian tube has a rim of *fimbria* (Latin for "fringe") that lies next to the ovary and is connected only by a thin muscular ligament. At the time of ovulation, this ligament contracts, pulling the flared end of the tube toward the ovary so it can receive the egg. Once tubebound, the egg coasts toward the uterus by the pulsing of the cilia, stopping as it reaches the narrowing section of the tube—about one-third of the way. This is the site where fertilization takes place and must occur within about a day of ovulation.

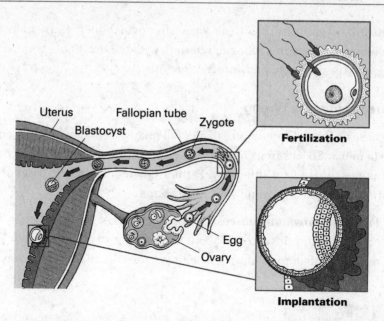

Uterus   Fallopian tube   Zygote

Blastocyst

Fertilization

Egg

Ovary

Implantation

From *The Merck Manual of Medical Information*, Second Home Edition, p. 1436, edited by Mark H. Beers. Copyright © 2003 by Merck & Co., Inc., Whitehouse Station, NJ. Available at: www.merck.com/mmhe.

After the egg is fertilized, it spends about three days in this end of the tube, where it divides and becomes two cells and then four cells and so on. The rich fluid within the tube nourishes the embryo. The beating cilia produce a current that allows the embryo to gently move to and fro, making slow progress toward the uterus, until it ultimately reaches the narrow, or *proximal,* end of the tube. By this time, the embryo is like a ball of cells with a partially fluid-filled center. Once deposited in the uterus, it begins implantation—this occurs around the 21st day of your

AN UNCOMMON EXPLANATION FOR "UNEXPLAINED INFERTILITY"

The fimbria needs a certain amount of freedom of movement in order to maneuver into position and successfully catch the egg at the time of ovulation. Some cases of unexplained infertility have been linked to a fallopian tube that is too close to the ovary and lacks this agility. One study found that in women with too short of a distance between the tube and the ovary—less than 2 cm—surgically freeing the end of the tube helped patients conceive without further treatment. This is an uncommon condition, but if you're planning on having a laparoscopy or any tubal surgery, ask your doctor to check for this—and fix it if you do have it.

menstrual cycle, or a little over a week after ovulation. It's easy to imagine how a blockage in a tube can interfere with the transit of sperm, egg, or embryo—and ultimately prevent pregnancy.

When Things Go Wrong

Because of the delicate nature of the fallopian tubes, they are susceptible to injury. So let's first consider the most common problems that contribute to tubal factor infertility. Farther down, I'll describe diagnostic tests and how to determine your tubal factor.

Pelvic inflammatory disease (PID) is the most common cause of tubal infertility, involved in about half of these cases. PID is an infection of the fallopian tubes, caused by a sexually transmitted disease

Case in Point

When I first met Anna, she was suffering from pelvic pain caused by scar tissue from a prior case of pelvic inflammatory disease, an infection resulting from a sexually transmitted disease. At 25, she had already had her left fallopian tube and ovary removed because of the scar tissue. Her right tube had also been operated on to release a large fluid collection. Before seeing me for the pain, she saw a physician who recommended a hysterectomy. Anna was single but hoping to have a family one day and was distraught over his advice.

I told Anna that I could perform surgery to remove any scar tissue and try to restore her fallopian tube to normal, but that I couldn't ensure that it would relieve her pain. I also made it clear that she would be at an elevated risk of developing an ectopic pregnancy—a pregnancy that implants prematurely in the fallopian tube rather than in the uterus. She decided to have the repair. At her six week follow-up, she said that her pelvic pain had improved. I encouraged her to use contraception until she decided she wanted to become pregnant.

About eight years passed before I saw Anna again. We bumped into each other at a local market. She told me that she stayed on contraception for the first three years of her marriage. Within three months of stopping, she conceived and had a little girl that was now three years old. Now she was pregnant again, just finishing her 12th week.

like gonorrhea or chlamydia. About 1 million women in the United States contract chlamydia each year, and at least half of them report later that they never knew they had it (the infection typically has no symptoms). PID can cause an obstruction at the distal end of the tube (nearest to the ovary), causing the tube to fill up with fluid, a condition called *hydrosalpinx.*

Salpingitis isthmica nodosa (SIN) is a common cause of proximal tubal obstruction. It is characterized by *diverticula,* saclike pouches that extend from the wall or the center of the tube. Over time, scarring develops and the tubal opening either narrows or becomes completely *occluded,* or blocked. A partially blocked tube increases the risk of ectopic pregnancy. SIN may be caused by inflammation or an infection. It should be treated before attempting fertility treatment.

Previous pelvic surgery is a known risk for tubal factor infertility. Surgery to the tube itself or even an adjacent organ like the appendix can affect the tube's delicate anatomy. If you've had surgical treatment of an ectopic pregnancy, the risk of your tube closing up is higher than if you've had a C-section or a simple laparoscopy, but it's highest if you've had a ruptured appendix or a pelvic abscess, as these surgeries have a high risk of postoperative infection.

ECTOPIC PREGNANCY

In about 1 percent of pregnancies, a fertile embryo will implant somewhere other than inside the womb. Over 90 percent of these ectopic pregnancies occur in the fallopian tube. Many things can contribute to the risk of developing an ectopic pregnancy, but the most common is a history of tubal disease, like PID, SIN, or having had any surgery to the tube. If you had an ectopic pregnancy, your chance of having another is 10 to 15 percent. If it's detected early, the tube can be saved and the ectopic tissue can be treated with a medication called methotrexate to prevent it from rupturing and creating a potentially life-threatening hemorrhage. I recommend all women have an ultrasound between the 5th and 7th week of pregnancy to confirm the location of the pregnancy early, before any symptoms of pain or bleeding occur. The test can save your tube and may even save your life.

TUBAL LIGATION FOR CONTRACEPTION

Nearly one in every four married women has had her "tubes tied," a misnomer for surgically blocking the fallopian tubes as a method of contraception. The most popular method of performing this minor procedure is using an electrocautery to burn and close up the tube, though this destroys about 1 to 2 cm of the tube. Other methods include clamps or clips, which may involve the destruction of a smaller section of tube, the removal of a section, or the removal of the entire tube. They are never, however, tied in a knot. Between 1 and 7 percent of women eventually choose to have a "reversal" of the tubal ligation. The chance of successful conception after a reversal depends on many factors, such as the method of the original surgery, the technique used for the reversal (the gold standard for reversal is doing it through microsurgery), and your age. If you're considering a reversal, obtain a copy of your medical record to see which method was used for your original procedure. See a board-certified reproductive endocrinologist to discuss the appropriateness of a tubal reversal versus IVF. See the website of the ASRM (www.asrm.org) for practice committee guidelines on tubal reconstruction. This information will facilitate your decision making.

Birth defects affecting the fallopian tubes are rare, but when they occur, infertility is usually the only symptom. When a birth defect is the result of a hormonal imbalance that occurred during fetal development, it often causes atrophy of one or both tubes. For example, early exposure to the potent estrogen diethylstilbestrol (DES), which may have been given to as many as 10 million women before it was banned in 1971, often resulted in tubal atrophy. Talk to your doctor if you think you may have been exposed to DES while in the womb, or have been told you have only one kidney (often a missing kidney and fallopian tube go hand in hand), or that you don't have both tubes. The degree of infertility and the treatment required varies depending on the severity of the structural deformity.

DIAGNOSTIC TESTS FOR TUBAL FACTOR

Although some people like to delay testing for tubal obstructions to save money, I recommend that everyone with infertility, with the exception of those with a very low risk of tubal factor, consider testing first.

The results will help determine the severity of your tubal factor and what treatments are most appropriate for you, saving you time and money in the end. There is overlap among these tests, so not all of them are necessary. Some of the less-expensive tests may, depending on the results, need to be confirmed by more involved and costly tests. Each has advantages and disadvantages, so weigh your options carefully. You are at very low risk of having a tubal factor if you have very mild menstrual cycles (with no cramping), no history of surgery, and no history of an STD. You may choose to forego testing and proceed with treatment, but if you don't conceive within three to six months, consider a more thorough evaluation for tubal factors. Once you decide which tests to take, enter your results into the "Tubal Factor Questionnaire" on page 180 to determine whether your tubes need to be factored in when considering treatment. Here are your options.

Chlamydia serology testing. I recommend that all women with infertility have a simple blood test for immune proteins to determine if they've ever had chlamydia—some fertility centers require it. An estimated 10 percent of women without any risk factors will test positive. If you're diagnosed with chlamydia, your health care provider will treat you and possibly your partner with antibiotics. Also consider having one of the imaging tests (below) to assess for any damage.

Hysterosalpingogram (HSG) is an imaging test using X-ray fluoroscopy. In this test, performed between the 3rd and 10th days of your menstrual cycle, your uterus and fallopian tubes are filled with

OIL AND WATER

Traditionally, an oil-based contrast called Lipiodol was used for all HSG studies. Over time, it was replaced with a water-based contrast that provided better images and had a lower risk of an allergic reaction. During the last decade, however, a growing number of studies have found that Lipiodol triples your chance of conceiving for about six months after it is administered. Although I typically use the water-based contrast, after I've confirmed that at least one tube is open, I'll inject 10 ml of Lipiodol and inform my patient that over the next six months, her chance of conception will be the highest. I suggest you request Lipiodol ahead of time unless you're allergic or have another contraindication.

Ask Dr. Greene

Q Is there any way to reduce the pain and discomfort of an HSG or sonohysterogram?

A These can be uncomfortable tests, but the pain can be minimized by taking the following precautions.

◆ Request a prescription for the topical anesthetic called EMLA (5 percent cream), as long you're not allergic. It's applied to the cervix by placing the cream in a cervical cap, like the contraceptive diaphragm, at least 30 minutes before your procedure—it's not systemically absorbed when used internally. This anesthetic will dramatically reduce or even eliminate pain. Women experienced at using the cervical cap for contraception are comfortable placing it at home before they go for their imaging study.

◆ Try to have the test performed by someone experienced at doing pelvic exams. Some radiologists, for example, don't do this intimate exam on a regular basis, so ask your OB or specialist to be present.

◆ Perform slow, deep-breathing exercises to lower your stress hormone and oxytocin levels—both hormones can heighten your sensitivity to pain.

◆ Take a set of headphones and listen to quiet music.

a contrast agent and an X-ray is taken. The radiologist watches to see if the fluid spills into the abdominal cavity (the radiation exposure is minimal). It can cause mild to moderate cramping. The HSG is reasonably accurate for detecting a proximal tubal blockage, but is much less precise for confirming distal tubal disease or scar tissue around the tubes. Have the images examined by both a radiologist and a trained fertility specialist, as each may interpret them differently. If you have an abnormal finding, you will need to take a more definitive test to determine if your tubes are patent (unobstructed). The HSG can be used for women with PID and birth defects, or to confirm the success of a tubal ligation reversal, as well as for other problems.

Sonohysterogram is my preferred imaging method, though not all doctors have the equipment. This test uses ultrasound instead of radiation, making it safer than HSG, somewhat more comfortable, and more cost effective since it can also provide images of your other reproductive organs at the same time. It can also be videotaped for review later. You may have to request prior to the test that the ultrasonographer uses Lipiodol to boost your chance of conception, once it's confirmed that your tubes are patent. If one or both tubes are occluded, you may need a laparoscopy to confirm a diagnosis. The sonohysterogram is used if you have had PID, SIN, birth defects, or previous pelvic surgery.

Laparoscopy with tubal dye study is considered the gold standard for making a diagnosis of tubal factor infertility because it involves direct visualization of all of the pelvic anatomy. But, it comes with the usual low risks of surgery and anesthesia, and, in many cases, you don't need it to get a diagnosis. It may be offered as a follow-up to an abnormal imaging test or can be done in conjunction with a laparoscopy you're having for another reason (such as to check for endometriosis). A laparoscopy is performed through one to four tiny incisions. A small amount of blue dye, called indigo carmine, is infused in your uterus as the surgeon watches it spill out of the fallopian tube into your abdomen. Once your tubes are confirmed patent, a small amount of Lipiodol may also be injected to boost your fertility—request this in advance of the procedure. Your doctor can also treat any scar tissue that may be restricting the ability of your tubes to move and function. Request that your doctor confirm that the fimbria—the flared end of your tube—appears normal and able to reach even the most distant site of ovulation on each ovary. If it's not, the end of the tube can be surgically freed to improve its mobility.

If you are considering having a laparoscopy, first see what other tests can be done through the laparoscopy at the same time (see chapters 9, 11, and 12) to improve your chance of success at the lowest possible financial cost. It's also a good idea to request that your doctor photograph your uterus, ovaries, and tubes, making a copy for you to retain for your medical records. This information can be invaluable if you later need to be seen by another specialist—it can save you another surgery.

See the Tubal Factor Questionnaire on page 180 and then record your tubal factor in the chart on page 226 to help determine what level treatment you may need to consider.

Tubal Factor 1: Presumed Fertile

There's no evidence that you have any tubal factor limiting your fertility. However, anyone can develop an ectopic pregnancy even without

TUBAL FACTOR QUESTIONNAIRE

Your tubal factor is based on the results of any of the diagnostic tests you've had as well as certain aspects of your reproductive history. Circle the answer that most accurately describes you or results of testing you've done. Total the scores for each answer and review your score below.

	0	1	2	3
My chlamydia serology is . . .	negative	never done	weak positive	positive
My HSG or sonohysterogram was . . .	normal	not done	equivocal	abnormal
My laparoscopy was . . .	normal	not done	mild findings	major findings
I've had pelvic surgery	Never	Yes, no infection	——	Yes, with infection
I've had a tubal ligation	No	Yes, but reversed	——	Yes
I've been exposed to DES	Never	Unknown	Suspected	Confirmed
I've had an ectopic pregnancy	Never	——	Once	Twice or more
I've been treated for STD's	Never	——	Once	Twice or more
I was born with [#] of kidneys	Two, I assume	——	One	——
I've been pregnant	Within 5 years	More than 5 years ago	Never	——

Total your score. Here's the bottom line:

Score	Severity
0–2:	Tubal factor 1
3–5:	Tubal factor 2
6–9:	Tubal factor 3
10 or more:	Tubal factor 4

any risk factors, so it's still a good idea to request an ultrasound within the first seven weeks of your pregnancy. At this level, you should base your treatment choices on other factors.

Tubal Factor 2: Mild

This mild level doesn't limit your fertility treatment options, but it should raise your awareness of this issue. I recommend that you consider a sono-hysterogram if you haven't had one already. If you choose to go right into fertility treatment (based upon your other factors), reexplore additional testing if you don't become pregnant within three to four treatment cycles. If you have tubal factor 2, you may have one of the following scenarios.

Unknown tubal patency. At least one of your tubes is assumed to be unobstructed. A more diagnostic test can confirm this, but you may decide to go right into fertility treatment.

Reversal of tubal ligation. If your reversal was successful, this won't present an obstacle for you. The best chance of a successful reversal is if it was performed by an experienced surgeon trained in microsurgical techniques. You'll still need frequent follow-ups to make sure that you don't develop an ectopic pregnancy.

History of ectopic pregnancy. If you've had an ectopic pregnancy and subsequently had a laparoscopy, HSG, or sonohysterogram confirming that your tubes are unobstructed, you can proceed with treatment as if your tubes were normal. But your risk of having another ectopic pregnancy is about 10 to 15 percent. Your risk of ectopic pregnancy can be increased further by certain BioMutagen exposures. So before you proceed, consider the following.

- *DES exposure* while in the womb increases your risk of having an ectopic pregnancy. If you're not sure whether you were exposed and you were born before 1971, when DES was banned, talk to a fertility specialist about your risk. You may have been exposed if your mother had a history of recurrent miscarriages or if a diagnostic test

Ask Dr. Greene

Q Should I consider having my fallopian tubes removed before having IVF?

A When fluid accumulates within the fallopian tube (a condition called a *hydrosalpinx*), it has been shown to hamper the ability of your uterus to support a pregnancy. Several studies have shown that surgically removing severely stretched and bloated tubes before proceeding with IVF improves pregnancy rates and dramatically lowers the risk of ectopic pregnancy. Studies have also found that instead of removing the tubes, occluding them at their proximal end with electrocautery may be equally as beneficial. Either procedure could improve your results.

finds that you have a T-shaped uterus (see chapter 11 for uterine factors). If you were exposed, it may be in your best interest to have your tubes occluded or removed and then proceed with IVF rather than risk another ectopic pregnancy.

◆ *Tobacco use* can increase your risk of having another ectopic pregnancy. The components of tobacco cause your body to convert estradiol into an antiestrogen, and some theorize that this loss of estrogen may hamper the ability of your tube to move the embryo along, causing it to implant prematurely there. If you're still smoking, this is another compelling reason to quit.

Successfully treated tubal disease. If you have been treated for tubal disease and your tubes are unobstructed, you have the freedom to choose from a large variety of treatment options. Just proceed cautiously, taking steps to ensure that you've minimized your risk of ectopic pregnancy. Reconsider your tubal factor if you don't conceive within three or four treatment cycles.

Tubal Factor 3: Moderate

You have significant tubal factor, but it may or may not have to be treated, depending on the specific damage to your tubes and its cause. In some cases, it might be better to work around your tubes and do IVF, since your eggs are withdrawn directly from your ovaries and do not have to traverse the tubes. But if you're going to pursue IVF, you may need to have your tubes removed to increase your chance for successful implantation. If you have tubal factor 3, you may have one of the following scenarios.

Previous tubal ligation was one of the original reasons that IVF was developed. Today, from a cost-benefit perspective, IVF is at least as successful as tubal reversal. If you'd like to consider a reversal, your success rate depends on the postoperative length of your tube as well as your other fertility factors. Your fertility specialist will need to assess whether at least 5 cm of the tube is salvageable. Any less is associated with a very low pregnancy rate even if your tubes are open.

Proximal tubal occlusion can be a difficult diagnosis to establish since this muscular portion of the tube can contract—giving the

Case in Point

Confident at the cause of her infertility, Sharon came to her consultation with me ready to schedule surgery. At 30, with two children, she had undergone a tubal ligation as a means of sterilization. Since then, she and her husband divorced. Now 38, she had recently married Jack, 42, who had fathered a child 15 years earlier. When Sharon and Jack came to see me, Sharon wanted me to "untie her tubes" to restore her fertility. I explained to them that even though they had both proven their fertility with previous partners, testing for ovarian reserve and a semen analysis were necessary to see if surgery was even worth considering. Their tests determined that Jack had male factor 1 and Sharon had ovarian factor 2. This means that all options, including reversal of Sharon's tubal ligation, were appropriate, but I still recommended they consider IVF instead.

When I saw their look of surprise, I explained that based upon Sharon's age, she had an increased chance of having twins, which they had informed me they wanted to try to avoid. By undergoing IVF, we could minimize their risk of having twins by only transferring one embryo and freezing the rest. The cost of an IVF cycle is typically less than the cost of a reversal of tubal ligation for women who don't have other factors that also need to be treated. Moreover, Sharon wouldn't have to worry about contraception after her pregnancy since her tubal ligation would still be functional. After careful consideration, they chose IVF. They produced five embryos, and we only transferred one. She became pregnant, and delivered a healthy boy just after her 39th birthday.

appearance of occlusion—only to relax later. Although there are procedures that attempt to open a proximal obstruction, they all have a high risk of failure, requiring repeat surgeries and carrying an elevated risk of ectopic pregnancy. I typically recommend IVF for women with confirmed proximal obstruction.

Distal tubal occlusion is the most variable factor, because your success rate depends on the severity of the blockage. About 25 percent of women with distal tubal disease have a mild-enough problem that surgery can correct the obstruction. Studies show that in those with mild occlusions, pregnancy rates approach 70 percent. However, if your HSG or sonohysterogram finds that your tube is dilated 2 cm or more, a sign of severe tubal disease, you should discuss the possibility of having your tubes removed.

Tubal Factor 4: Severe

Your tubal factor is severe enough to limit your treatment options to IVF. Before you do so, however, it's important to identify your other fertility factors so that your prognosis can be accurately assessed. You may even want to consider an interval procedure to have your fallopian tubes removed, since doing so may improve your success rate with IVF.

◆ ◆ ◆

Severe tubal factor was once an end-of-the-line diagnosis for women. Since the birth of the first baby through IVF in 1978, however, severe tubal factor became just another aspect of what needs to be considered in developing a treatment plan. Yet, you and your partner need to carefully consider which options are most appropriate. It's important that you feel comfortable asking questions about risks, benefits, and success rates with every option you consider.

11 Uterine Factor

Your last stop on your way to pregnancy is your uterus, where implantation takes place and where your baby will reside for nearly 280 days. Uterine factor, which typically leads to a failure to implant or miscarriage, is estimated to contribute to 5 to 10 percent of infertility cases. I believe this is an underestimate, but because doctors perceive that there's a low risk of uterine factor, it's often overlooked. Another reason uterine factor is under diagnosed is that it typically doesn't become apparent until after conception; many women with uterine problems aren't initially viewed as infertile because they do become pregnant—but then they miscarry because of the uterine factor. Often, the evaluation of this factor is delayed or missed entirely. I believe that a subtle, undiagnosed uterine factor is a critical yet overlooked element for many couples given the diagnosis of "unexplained infertility."

Failure to implant is not a rare event. Of all pregnancies in all couples in which an embryo travels down the fallopian tubes and makes it into the uterus, about half are lost because of a failure to implant. Most of these losses occur early enough in the process that a woman never even knows she was pregnant. I try to save my patients from having to endure an early pregnancy loss by considering in advance the anatomical factors that might contribute to implantation failure. Such factors include fibroids, polyps, adhesions, and malformations. But the vast

THE HORMONE PLAYERS

◆ **Estradiol** begins to rise early in the cycle as the eggs enter the last stage of their development. It starts to prepare the uterus early for implantation by promoting proliferation of the uterine lining.

◆ **Progesterone** production begins after ovulation and stops further growth of the uterine lining, but promotes its maturation into a fertile ground for implantation.

◆ **Human chorionic gonadotropin (HCG)** The embryo produces HCG to signal the granulosa cells in the ovary to increase the production of estradiol and progesterone as the pregnancy develops.

◆ **Insulin** plays a vital role in regulating energy metabolism of the endometrial cells as well as rendering them more sensitive to progesterone.

◆ **Prolactin** is one of the first hormones detected in the uterus at the time of implantation. Produced by the developing embryo, this hormone plays a critical role in maintaining the balance of electrolytes within the gestational sac in which your baby will grow.

majority of implantation failures occur because of underlying hormonal imbalance, which often leads to miscarriage (see chapter 12 for information on preventing recurrent miscarriages).

THE WINDOW OF IMPLANTATION

After an egg is fertilized and the embryo travels down your fallopian tube into your uterus, it must implant into the endometrium, the lining of your uterus. Every month, your endometrium undergoes a transformation from a thin unfertile lining to a lush fertile environment. These changes are orchestrated by your hormones. The developing follicle produces estradiol, which fuels the growth of the endometrium, and also promotes the differentiation of endometrial cells into at least 18 types of specialized ones—for instance, some serve immune function, others provide nourishment, and others help the embryo attach to the lining. Estradiol also enhances blood flow to the endometrium.

Following ovulation, the follicle cells that were left behind, specifically the granulosa cells, receive a signal in the form of HCG to begin producing progesterone from cholesterol. The cells become so engorged with cholesterol that they take on a yellowish color, earning them their name corpus luteum, Latin for "yellowish body." Progesterone is considered a key pregnancy hormone because it helps prevent the overgrowth of the endometrium and helps the endometrial cells mature into their specialized functions that promote implantation and support the pregnancy. It also dampens the immune system so that white blood cells don't mistake the embryo for a foreign body.

About seven days after ovulation, the endometrium is primed to receive the embryo—if an egg was fertilized—opening a *window of implantation* that lasts for about 72 hours. The embryo is encased within a tough protective membrane called the *zona pellucida.* Within three days of arrival into the uterus, the embryo will hatch from this shell and attach to the uterine wall. The endometrial cells have specialized

Ask Dr. Greene

Q Can the embryo fall out of my uterus when it arrives?

A This is something many women think about, but confess they feel silly asking. Fertility specialists used to ask the same question, which prompted us to place our patients on bed rest after an embryo was placed in their wombs during an IVF procedure. We now know that after ovulation you have subtle contractions that begin in the lower uterus and move upward, acting as a gentle pressure that keeps the egg aloft, giving it time to implant. There are several other safeguards in place: chemical bonds similar to static electricity, sticky proteins, and hairlike structures that keep the embryo clinging to the endometrium until implantation takes place.

TOO MUCH INSULIN MAY INTERFERE WITH IMPLANTATION

Fertility specialists have long known that women with PCOS have a higher miscarriage rate than other women. Only recently has it become apparent that insulin is responsible for this risk. When insulin is too high, as it is in women with PCOS, it tips the balance of estradiol to testosterone in favor of testosterone, making the endometrial cells less receptive to implantation. Lowering insulin levels by taking the insulin-sensitizing drug metformin can help restore this balance. One large study published in 2006 demonstrated that when nondiabetic women with PCOS continued taking metformin during pregnancy, the miscarriage rate dropped from 36 percent to 11 percent. If you have PCOS, talk to your health care provider about continuing metformin after you've conceived.

structures and proteins that hold the embryo in place until implantation is completed, typically about 10 days after ovulation.

Ask Dr. Greene

Q Does it matter if I have a "tipped uterus"?

A For many years, it was believed that if a woman's uterus was retroverted or "tipped backward," she would have difficulty conceiving. This conclusion was drawn because problems like endometriosis or scarring, which can cause infertility, can also cause the uterus to tip backward toward the spine. The disorders were the cause of the infertility, not the orientation of the uterus. Many women are simply born with a tipped uterus. As a pregnancy progresses, the uterus will straighten up and orient toward a woman's head rather than her spine.

DIAGNOSING UTERINE FACTOR

Everybody should think about getting tested for uterine factor, especially if you need imaging tests to diagnose other factors. Testing should focus on either the anatomical structure of the uterus, including such problems as fibroids, adhesions, and uterine malformations, or on its functioning. As I mentioned, hormones that can affect implantation and cause miscarriage are discussed in the recurrent miscarriage section in chapter 12. Below, I review the most common tests offered and how useful they are. Some providers order outdated tests because they're familiar with them, even though current research shows that they're inaccurate or misleading. On the other hand, many doctors offer tests that are so new as to still be considered experimental.

Hydrosonography (sonohysterogram). As I've mentioned, this is my preferred test, especially if you're having other factors assessed simultaneously. A sonohysterogram is an ultrasound performed while placing a small amount of sterile saline within the uterine chamber to inflate the uterus in order to visualize the shape, size, and presence of any abnormalities. This procedure can be performed at most fertility centers with little or no discomfort.

Hysterosalpingogram (HSG) This imaging study often ordered to look for tubal patency can also provide useful information about uterine anatomy—but only when performed properly. Too often, our story

Robert: When our doctor recommended that Morgan do a hydrosonography, we ultimately decided against it. Though she worried about her uterine factor, she was clearly at low risk because she had become pregnant once (she miscarried at six weeks), and she did not have any risk factors like previous infections, surgery, or pain. We decided that at this point additional testing was not warranted, though we'd consider it in the future. We decided to live with the uncertainty of not knowing for sure. For Morgan, this decision gave her some sense of control in the treatment process.

sloppy techniques such as leaving a speculum (an instrument inserted to reveal your cervix) in the vagina during the examination or placing the instruments too deeply into the cervix obscures much of the image. This test involves placing contrast material into the uterus via a small catheter inserted through the cervix, and taking X-ray images at several intervals. If performed correctly, this is not a bad test, though it can cause discomfort. I still prefer the sonohysterogram if it is available.

Hysteroscopy. Although this outpatient procedure is considered the most definitive method for evaluating a woman's uterus, it is also the most costly and invasive. I generally reserve this test for patients that had an abnormal sonohysterogram or HSG, or are undergoing another surgical procedure like a laparoscopy. Under anesthesia, a small amount of air or saline is placed into the uterus and then a slender, telescope-like instrument is inserted through the cervix to view the inside chamber of the uterus. The doctor can also take biopsies or remove small polyps or fibroids during this procedure.

DETERMINING YOUR UTERINE FACTOR

Because most women with a uterine factor won't have any symptoms, a questionnaire isn't helpful to determine your factor level. Instead, the results of your imaging study will indicate which category you fall into. Read all of the categories to see if you have any of the conditions that characterize each level. If you have never had a successful pregnancy (one without complications) and choose to delay testing, then I suggest

DIAGNOSTIC TESTS TO AVOID

◆ **Postcoital test.** This decades-old test has been deemed invalid since at least 1990, but somehow remains part of the workup at many fertility clinics today. The postcoital test, which I described in detail on page 144, involves taking a Pap smear–type sample from the woman shortly after intercourse to look for motile sperm in the cervical mucus. The research reveals that the test frequently leads to more tests and treatments, but has no value in predicting pregnancy rates. Don't waste your time or money.

◆ **Endometrial biopsy.** This 50-year-old test was described as "worse than useless; it is misleading," in a recent review. For this procedure, a woman has a small biopsy of the uterine lining around day 21 of her menstrual cycle to examine how well primed it is for implantation. But because hormones shift from month to month, doctors need to perform this test three months in a row to achieve any semblance of accuracy. This adds cost and discomfort and creates a delay in treatment. I emphatically recommend against this test.

◆ **E-tegrity Test.** This is a modification of the endometrial biopsy. The biopsy tissue is also tested for a protein called *beta 3 integrin,* which is involved in embryo attachment to the endometrium. This combination may provide useful recommendations for improving treatment outcome, but it's so new that I'm waiting for more research that confirms its role before I recommend this expensive test for my patients.

you approach the treatment section assuming that you have uterine factor 2, until proven otherwise. That will draw your attention back to clarifying this issue further if you are not quickly successful with other fertility treatments. Record your uterine factor in the chart on page 226 to help determine what level treatment you may need to consider.

Uterine Factor 1: Presumed Fertile

Your uterus is probably normal and should not impact your treatment choices. But the hormone environment within your uterus changes on a month to month basis as levels of progesterone, estradiol, testosterone, and insulin vary. After you get pregnant, review the section on recurrent miscarriages (page 209) to determine what hormonal tests you might need to ensure that your endometrium is getting what it needs to carry your baby to term. You likely fit into one of these two scenarios.

Untested, but had a previous pregnancy. If you've been pregnant without complications like preterm labor, an infection of the uterus, or surgery, such as a cesarean section, you don't have uterine factor. If not, it is worth considering an imaging study if no other fertility factor emerges to explain your difficulty conceiving.

Normal imaging study. If you've had an imaging study confirm that there is no anatomical problem, then you're in the clear.

Uterine Factor 2: Mild

Your imaging test has revealed a minor problem. Your specific diagnosis will determine what should be done about your uterine factor. Here are the most common problems that cause mild factor.

Small fibroids. About 20,000 surgeries are performed in the United States per year to remove uterine fibroids, benign tumors made of muscle fibers and connective collagen embedded in the wall of the uterus. This high rate of surgery prompted the ASRM to publish guidelines recommending against surgical removal of fibroids that aren't causing symptoms like excessive bleeding or pain, unless they are causing a distortion in the uterus. ASRM also tried to quell the unjustified fear among physicians that small fibroids will grow during a pregnancy and interfere with a vaginal delivery. Several studies have found that although they can grow slightly in the first trimester of pregnancy, they often revert back to their original size or even become smaller before delivery. The bottom line: your treatment should not be affected by your fibroids if they're small, not causing symptoms, and aren't changing the shape or size of your uterus. Ask your doctor to document their size and location during any ultrasound exam for future comparison.

Mild uterine adhesions. The uterus is lined with a film of cells called the *basal layer,* which regenerates the lush layers of endometrial cells to prepare for implantation each month. If this layer is damaged— either through infection or previous surgery—gaps can occur in the fertile endometrium. When this occurs, the area typically heals by forming a scar called an *adhesion,* where no endometrial cells grow. In an imaging test, it would appear as a "filling defect" or a disruption in the flow of the testing fluid. If you have this finding, a hysteroscopy may be recommended to clarify whether adhesions are present. Adhesions are typically removed during the hysteroscopy and no further treatment is necessary.

Uterine polyps. These are benign cauliflower-shaped growths that are composed of endometrial cells. They are a common source of abnormal uterine bleeding, but their role in fertility is uncertain. They appear on a sonohysterogram or an HSG as a discrete filling defect. Since they are easily removed by hysteroscopy, I recommend you do so prior to having infertility treatment. They can also be removed through a procedure called a *dilation and curettage* (D & C), which involves widening the cervical opening and then gently scraping the wall of the uterus to remove the polyp. The advantage of hysteroscopy over a D & C is that it allows removal of the polyp under direct visualization without damaging the adjacent tissue and risking new adhesions. If you choose to have a D & C, using a BioIdentical estradiol or a birth control pill postsurgery can help reduce the risk of adhesions forming.

Arcuate uterus. The uterus is normally shaped like an inverted triangle. But in this most common form of uterine malformation, there is a small indentation in the top central portion of this triangle, making the uterine chamber appear more heart-shaped. An arcuate uterus does not warrant any treatment whatsoever, and will not affect your fertility. So if you see this description on the imaging report, don't let it affect your treatment choices.

Uterine Factor 3: Moderate

As a result of a congenital problem or a growth like fibroids, your uterus has an abnormal shape that may be impacting your ability to conceive, or, more typically, affecting your ability to carry a pregnancy. Discuss with your doctor whether your specific uterine malformation can be corrected. If not, it can typically be managed as part of your treatment plan.

Large uterine fibroids. As a woman ages, her risk of developing fibroids increases as does the size of the fibroids. By their late 30s, about 20 to 50 percent of women have fibroids (the range depends on race; it's most common in women of African descent and least common in Asian women). As fibroids grow, they're more likely to bleed or cause complications. If you have fibroids large enough to cause abnormal bleeding or pain, or to alter the shape of your uterine cavity, the ASRM recommends that they be surgically removed and

Case in Point

Adrianna made an appointment to see me after already having a second opinion confirming that she should have a hysterectomy—surgery to remove her uterus—because she had large fibroids. At 33 and without any children, Adrianna considered this a last-resort option. After reviewing her records and confirming her diagnosis, I reassured her that she had other options—either a myomectomy or an embolization. Because Adrianna had at least seven fibroids, I recommended a myomectomy. She agreed.

In preparation for her surgery, I placed Adrianna on a BioLimited hormone, Synarel, to shrink the fibroids. I also gave her a low dose of estradiol—the Climara patch—to reduce symptoms like hot flashes that the Synarel might cause. After three months, Adrianna's uterus had shrunk in size by about a third and she was ready for surgery. Her operation took nearly four hours. Just prior to completing her surgery, I carefully wrapped her uterus in a material called INTERCEED that would dissolve within a few weeks, but would reduce the chance that she would form scar tissue. I confirmed that both fallopian tubes were patent as well. I placed Adrianna on a birth control pill, Yaz, to promote healing by rapidly restoring her estrogen and progestin levels as well as provide contraception during her recovery. She also stopped the Synarel.

After two months, I encouraged Adrianna to stop the birth control pill and use the OV-Watch to identify her most fertile period and boost her chances of conceiving. The very next month, she conceived. Her pregnancy was complicated by mild preterm labor, which was treated with progesterone to promote uterine relaxation. At 39 weeks, she delivered a baby boy by cesarean section. Due to the extensive surgery on her uterus, I advised against labor and vaginal delivery—a standard recommendation.

the uterine muscle repaired through a bikini incision in a procedure called a *myomectomy.* You may be given a BioAntagonist hormone prior to surgery to temporarily create a menopause-like estrogen deficiency, which in turn shrinks the fibroids, typically by 10 to 30 percent. BioAntagonists are not recommended instead of surgery because they do not improve fertility alone. There is also a new, less-invasive procedure, called *fibroid embolization,* in which a catheter is inserted through a vein in the thigh to obstruct the blood vessels that feed the fibroids, depriving them of the oxygen and nutrition they need to thrive. Large studies have not been performed to determine the impact of this new procedure on future fertility. This should only be considered on a case-by-case basis. If you'd like to consider this less-invasive option, talk to your doctor about whether you're a good candidate for it.

Severe uterine adhesions. Women with moderate to severe adhesions often report light menstrual flow because sections of the uterine lining are replaced by scar tissue and have poor blood flow. Studies show that about 15 percent of women that have a D & C develop adhesions. If your sonohysterogram or HSG detected a filling defect, and you have a history of either light menstrual cycles or D & C procedures, see a reproductive endocrinologist or a gynecologist experienced in hysteroscopy to remove the adhesions. You'll likely want to wait at least one or two menstrual cycles after surgery before moving forward with fertility treatment. I recommend you use birth control pills after your surgery to promote healing.

Uterine malformations. During the first month of embryo development, males and females develop a pair of tubelike structures called *Müllerian* ducts along the developing spinal column in an area called the *gonadal ridge.* In females, *anti-Müllerian hormone (AMH)* is absent during the first trimester, resulting in the fusion of these Müllerian ducts and the atrophy of the wall between them to form one uterus with two fallopian tubes. (In males, AMH is present during early fetal development, producing the vas deferens while causing the Müllerian ducts to atrophy.) If the wall between the Müllerian ducts in females doesn't atrophy or only partly atrophies, which occurs in about 2 to 3 percent of all women, it results in a variety of uterine defects. These defects either block the necessary blood supply to support a pregnancy or inhibit the ability of the uterus to grow rapidly enough to accommodate the growth of the developing baby. These defects can be caused by exposure during fetal development to BioMutagens such as DES and thalidomide or by exposure to certain infections like rubella. About 7 percent of the women with uterine malformations may also have a genetic cause that can be passed down to their daughters. You may wish to discuss this with a genetic counselor. First, let's consider how each anomaly impacts your ability to carry a pregnancy. If you've had a sonohysterogram or HSG

Case in Point

Alena was referred to me after she had a miscarriage and it was discovered during an ultrasound that she had a very small uterus. Her menstrual cycles had been normal, and she and her husband had only recently begun trying to conceive.

I scheduled a sonohysterogram to more clearly visualize the shape and size of her uterus and to determine the status of her fallopian tubes. The results suggested she had a *unicornuate uterus*—a long, cylindrical-shaped uterus with only one fallopian tube. I explained that this may have contributed to her pregnancy loss. Although she did have both ovaries, this test would not allow me to visualize whether her other fallopian tube was present. I recommended a magnetic resonance imaging (MRI) test, which confirmed she had only one fallopian tube and one kidney (women with one fallopian tube are at risk of having only one kidney, too). I counseled her that nothing further should be done except to monitor her more closely during her next pregnancy to reduce the chance for another miscarriage. I reassured her that most women with this condition can carry a pregnancy successfully, but that they are at higher risk of preterm delivery. Alena and her husband decided to use an ovulation kit to conceive, and we agreed that if they weren't successful within a year, they'd return to discuss fertility treatment.

Less than a year later, I got a call from Alena telling me that she was pregnant. I performed an early ultrasound and confirmed that the pregnancy was located within her long, slender uterus. Since her progesterone level was a bit low, I gave her some progesterone to reduce the chance of a miscarriage. She delivered a healthy boy.

that is suggestive of an anomaly, you may need an MRI to diagnose which malformation you have.

• *Partial uterine septum,* a wall partially dividing the uterus, is associated with the highest risk of first trimester miscarriage. But it is also the easiest problem to treat. Since the "partition" tends to have poor blood flow, it can easily be removed by surgery to create one larger uterine chamber. Studies suggest that correcting a uterine septum can improve your chance of delivering a baby about fourfold. Ask your doctor about his experience in correcting this problem—you'll improve your chances of success if the surgeon is an experienced reproductive surgeon.

- *Unicornuate uterus* is a long, cylindrical-shaped uterus ending in only one fallopian tube. This is the least common of uterine anomalies, and its affect on pregnancy is not well documented. Based on the existing research, women with this anomaly have a higher risk of second trimester miscarriage and preterm birth. They also have a higher risk of infertility—impacting about one in four women with this problem—likely due to compromised blood flow to the ovaries and uterus. There is no treatment recommended for a unicornuate uterus except for careful surveillance during pregnancy by an OB who specializes in high-risk pregnancies.

- *Bicornuate uterus* is a uterus that is Y-shaped instead of triangular. This "Y" results from the incomplete fusion of the Müllerian ducts—like a zipper than isn't closed completely—creating one cervix leading to two separate uterine chambers (the arms of the Y), each ending in its own fallopian tube. This can only be detected by an imaging study, and if you have this defect, you will have a fairly good pregnancy rate, but with an elevated risk of preterm delivery. There is no treatment recommended, except for careful surveillance during pregnancy by a high-risk OB.

- *Didelphic uterus.* When the Müllerian ducts fail to unite at all, a woman will have two elongated uteruses, each with a cervix and a fallopian tube. In some cases, one uterus is more completely formed or may have a more normal fallopian tube, or one uterus is atrophied. You would know if you have a didelphic uterus if you've ever had a pelvic exam, as it's something your doctor can detect during an examination with a speculum. In fact, your doctor should be performing two Pap smears, one for each cervix, during your annual exams. A didelphic uterus does not require any specific treatment, but you have a slightly higher risk of preterm delivery if you have one. It can typically be managed by close surveillance during your pregnancy. If you are undergoing intrauterine insemination (see chapter 13), discuss with your doctor the health of each uterus and whether one or both should be inseminated.

Uterine Factor 4: Severe

At this level, your uterine factor can't be resolved or corrected. One option you'll need to consider is a gestational surrogate—having another

CHECK YOUR KIDNEYS

Between the 8th and 10th week of fetal development, the uterus, the fallopian tubes, and the tubes that flow from the kidneys to the bladder, called ureters, form from a pair of parallel tube-shaped structures. That's why 75 percent of women with uterine anomalies also have eccentrically located ureters. If you have a uterine anomaly, you should request an imaging study, such as an intravenous pyelogram (IVP) or magnetic resonance imaging (MRI) study, to locate the ureters. It's important to know where they are if you need a cesarean section, to prevent accidentally damaging them during the surgery. The kidney usually functions normally.

woman carry the pregnancy and deliver your baby. In chapter 14, I'll describe how to incorporate this into your treatment plan. Here are the most common conditions that cause uterine factor 4.

Absent uterus

- *Hysterectomy.* In the United States, about 600,000 hysterectomies are performed each year; about one-third of these procedures are performed to treat uterine fibroids. Some women come to regret this decision when they decide they want to have a child. Although uterine transplantation has been considered by

UTERINE TRANSPLANT

There are very few physical and medical obstacles to having a uterine transplant for women who have undergone a hysterectomy but had previously frozen embryos. The uterus is a very simple organ that doesn't wear out like the ovaries or some other body parts, and instead just passively responds to the hormones that stimulate it. The real obstacles are ethical in nature. Though this procedure has not yet been performed (as of the printing of this book), this is most likely to be the first type of reproductive transplant using a deceased person's organ. Transplants have been done for other reproductive organs, like the ovaries, but only between live twin sisters. Nonetheless, ethics boards have condoned the procedure, concluding that a uterine transplant is a valid and ethically acceptable procedure. It's only a matter of time until the first woman with a uterine transplant delivers a healthy baby.

researchers, transplant surgeons, and ethic boards, it is not yet available. The only treatment option is the use of a surrogate (see chapter 14).

◆ *Congenital absence.* A small fraction of women are born without a uterus. If you fall into this category, a test for ovarian reserve is essential before considering whether you want to use a surrogate with your own embryo, since you may be at risk of premature ovarian failure as well, and not have healthy eggs. In addition, you may want to speak to a genetic counselor, since nearly 10 percent of women born without a uterus have a genetic cause for this birth defect that can be passed down to their daughter.

Previous endometrial ablation. A growing number of procedures are being marketed to women with heavy vaginal bleeding. These procedures use electricity, a laser, heat, or cold to damage the basal layer of the endometrium, permanently preventing it from regenerating each month in response to your hormones. The result is a dramatic reduction or complete elimination of menstrual flow. Unfortunately, it also means that there is no place for an embryo to implant. Women that have undergone an endometrial ablation still have their uterus but cannot carry a pregnancy. Women are not always told that this causes permanent sterilization, as some doctors may assume a woman is not interested in future pregnancies. Surrogacy is the only treatment option.

◆ ◆ ◆

Often uterine factors aren't considered until after a woman has had three or more consecutive miscarriages—these will be covered in the next chapter. Whether you are tested before undergoing treatment, it's important to reevaluate your uterine factor if your treatments are not successful.

12

Endometriosis and Recurrent Miscarriage

You have two more fertility factors to consider before moving on to treatment: endometriosis and recurring miscarriages. Neither of these may apply to you, but if one does, it could be the primary obstacle in your quest to deliver a healthy baby. Your fertility specialist will be very familiar with each problem, but by educating yourself about them, you'll be able to guide your doctor in deciding which tests and treatments to use.

ENDOMETRIOSIS

As many as 20 to 50 percent of women with infertility have *endometriosis*—a condition in which the endometrial cells that normally line the uterus migrate to other locations in their body. Of all reproductive-age women, 10 to 15 percent have the disorder, which was once limited to women in their later reproductive years, but is increasingly being seen in teens and young women.

Endometriosis can cause a range of symptoms, including infertility, pain before and during periods, pain during sex and urination, and constipation or diarrhea. But keep in mind that not all women with endometriosis have infertility or any of these symptoms. Once the endometrial cells spread to their new sites—most commonly on the outside surfaces of the uterus, the fallopian tubes, the ovaries, the bladder, or

---

THE HORMONE PLAYERS

◆ **Estradiol.** Endometrial cells lining the uterus convert testosterone to estradiol, which then fuels their own growth, but cells of women with endometriosis do this more efficiently, suggesting that endometriosis cells proliferate more rapidly.

◆ **Progesterone** limits the growth of endometrial cells by making them less sensitive to estradiol's growth-promoting effects. The high progesterone levels experienced during pregnancy provide a protective effect against developing endometriosis, and can induce a remission in women that have it at the onset of pregnancy.

◆ **Oxytocin** promotes contractions of the uterus. There is evidence that women with endometriosis produce more oxytocin than other women, possibly explaining why they tend to have severe menstrual cramps.

---

the colon—they act as seeds that grow into clusters or lesions. Here, these cells continue to respond to the monthly hormonal signals to proliferate and shed as if they were still lining the uterus. But since they cannot be shed in their new locations, they instead cause bleeding, swelling, and scar tissue. Endometriosis can also occur within the ovary, a condition known as an *endometrioma.*

It is not known why some women develop endometriosis and others don't. Endometriosis is like a jigsaw puzzle. We've identified many and maybe all of the pieces. But figuring out exactly how they fit together is an ongoing challenge. Here's some of what we know so far.

Retrograde menstruation. Though it has long been debated, the prevailing explanation behind the spread of endometrial cells is what's called retrograde menstruation. Just as the name implies, uterine contractions force menstrual blood containing endometrial cells up through the fallopian tubes and into the pelvis, rather than down toward the vagina and out of your body. The uterus has different types of normal contractions, and the type that causes retrograde menstruation is one that moves about halfway up the uterus—this specialized contraction is thought to help keep an embryo from dropping too quickly out of the uterus, giving it time to implant. Some evidence suggests that women with endometriosis experience this type of contraction excessively and at inappropriate times. These contractions could also explain the higher incidence of pelvic pain in women with endometriosis.

Genetics. Endometriosis tends to run in families, as do certain traits that predispose you to this condition. The significance of the genetic link is not yet known, but as we learn more, it may provide a key to preventing or treating endometriosis more effectively in the future.

Immunological factors. Women with endometriosis are more likely to have immune problems like allergies and asthma, as well as autoimmune diseases such as rheumatoid arthritis, multiple sclerosis, and lupus. Some research suggests that in rare instances, when endometrial cells are found in distant sites, a weakened immune system might have allowed them to spread through the lymph or blood systems.

BioMutagens. Numerous studies have revealed a strong link between exposure to certain BioMutagens and the risk of developing endometriosis. Two common hormone-disrupting pollutants—

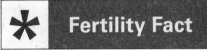

Fertility Fact

The Origins of Retrograde Menstruation

Studies comparing endometriosis sufferers to controls have found that retrograde menstruation occurs in between 60 and 98 percent of *all* women. Whenever a finding is that prevalent, there is typically a potential health benefit. It's widely believed that retrograde menstruation prevents anemia. For our ancestors, the oxygen-carrying mineral iron was not as easily obtained in their food as it is today. The amount of iron women lose in their menstrual flow can clearly lead to anemia if it's not replaced. Retrograde menstruation gives your body the ability to retain and recycle this mineral instead of losing it through menstruation. Today, it's an unnecessary adaptation, since iron is easily obtained through food.

THE RED-HAIR FACTOR

A few studies have reported that redheads had a higher risk of endometriosis than others; one study found the risk was doubled. The connection between the two seemingly unrelated conditions can be traced back to a specific chromosome. The gene that's responsible for red hair is located on chromosome number 19, the same chromosome responsible for several immune functions. This provides a plausible explanation for why women with an alteration to this chromosome may experience both red hair and a higher risk for immunologic problems.

dioxin and phthalates—demonstrate the strongest and most direct link. Dioxins, present primarily in animal fats, can cause shifts in thyroid hormones and act as potent estrogens by binding to receptors and promoting the growth of endometrial cells.

Phthalates are found in numerous consumer products, but nail polish is perhaps the greatest source of exposure for women. They are also created in our food when cooking in plastic containers in microwave ovens. Phthalates can cause an imbalance between testosterone and estrogen that can boost the growth of errant endometrial cells.

Research found that women who ate a diet high in green vegetables had a 70 percent reduced risk of developing endometriosis. Those who had a high fruit intake had a 40 percent reduced risk. In contrast, those whose diet was high in beef and ham—in which dioxins are often prevalent—had double the risk of recurrence. Also, avoid products packaged in recyclable #3 plastics or cling wraps—and don't microwave in plastics. To learn how to reduce your exposure further, visit the website of the Endometriosis Association, a nonprofit group that has funded much of the research on pollutants (www.endometriosisassn.org).

> **Did you know ?**
>
> The current medical research confirms that following dietary recommendations like those in my Perfect Balance Fertility Program may reduce your risk of a recurrence of endometriosis.

ENDOMETRIOSIS AND FERTILITY

About half of all women with endometriosis have infertility. Though there are strong associations between the two conditions, a cause-and-effect relationship has not been definitively established. Based on the latest research, here are some ways that endometriosis may be reducing your chances of pregnancy.

Pain during sex. Three out of four women with endometriosis report pain, especially during sexual intercourse. For some women, the pain becomes so intense around the time of ovulation that sex is out of the question, an obvious barrier to natural conception.

ADENOMYOSIS: A GROWING FERTILITY CHALLENGE

When endometrial cells burrow deep into the muscular wall of the uterus, it is called *adenomyosis,* a condition that causes chronic pelvic pain or heavy menstrual bleeding. Sometimes called "endometriosis of the uterine muscle," adenomyosis is more common in women who've gone through labor and delivery or have had surgical procedures like a D & C. But because of diet and exposure to BioMutagens, it is increasingly being seen in women in their late 30s or early 40s who are trying to become pregnant for the first time and had no prior surgery. In these women, studies show that adenomyosis tends to disrupt the useful contractions that propel sperm toward the fallopian tubes, perhaps contributing to infertility. If you have severe pelvic pain or menstrual cramps, talk to your doctor about whether you should have a high-resolution ultrasound or an MRI to check for adenomyosis.

Inhibited sperm transport. Although the type of contraction that promotes retrograde menstruation (and is thought to keep an embryo suspended in the uterus) is more vigorous in women with endometriosis, the type of contraction that propels sperm toward the ovulating ovary tends to be weaker. It is yet to be proven, but this may slow the journey of sperm, which can be especially important if your partner has diminished sperm function.

Altered immune function. Women with endometriosis tend to have more fluid surrounding their ovaries. This fluid contains active immune cells, which may attack sperm or the ovulated egg. In addition, some sufferers form antibodies against the errant cells. But these antibodies can also attack the normal endometrial cells within the uterus and interfere with implantation.

Inflammation. Endometriosis can create inflammation around the fallopian tubes. When this happens, the fimbria on the end of the tubes swell and become less effective at capturing an egg as it's released. The tube can also become impaired in other subtle ways, as evidenced by the higher rate of ectopic pregnancies in endometriosis sufferers.

Scar tissue. As endometriosis begins to heal, scar tissue can form. If it causes a kink or blockage in the fallopian tube, it can prevent the

IRRITABLE BOWEL SYNDROME (IBS) AND INTERSTITIAL CYSTITIS (IC)

Women with endometriosis are at greater risk of episodes of constipation, diarrhea, or both, called *irritable bowel syndrome (IBS)*. They are also at risk of recurrent irritation of the bladder, called *interstitial cystitis (IC)*. The reproductive organs, the digestive tract, and the bladder all share common nerve pathways, increasing the chance that signals can get crossed so that pain originating in one system will contribute to pain in the other, or simply be perceived as pain in the other. Evidence suggests that this nerve sharing creates a hypersensitization among neighboring organs. If you have IBS or IC, and have infertility trouble, consider being evaluated for endometriosis. Or, if you have endometriosis that has been treated, but your symptoms haven't improved, request an evaluation for IBS or IC to fully restore your quality of life.

sperm and egg from ever crossing paths. Sometimes sheetlike scar tissue, called *adhesions,* can form over the ovary and prevent the egg from reaching the tube after it's released.

DIAGNOSING ENDOMETRIOSIS

Testing is required to determine if you have endometriosis and its impact on your fertility. If you have pelvic pain that is significant enough to impair your quality of life, I recommend that you be examined. When endometriosis is treated, it can reduce your pain dramatically. A laparoscopy, the minimally invasive procedure performed under anesthesia and using tiny incisions, is the only appropriate way to diagnose endometriosis. A laparoscopy allows the surgeon to visualize endometriosis lesions and to surgically remove *(ablate)* them. I highly recommend that you request that your surgeon document the extent of your endometriosis, a standardized process called *staging,* using ASRM criteria. The ASRM created a staging sheet (available at www.asrm.org) in order to help surgeons characterize a woman's endometriosis as well as to improve communication among fertility specialists. Using the staging sheet, the surgeon simply places marks on the drawings to identify the location, size, and depth of the lesions. Each lesion is then scored. The total score indicates the severity of your endometriosis and

ENDOMETRIOSIS RISK ASSESSMENT

This questionnaire will provide you with an estimate of your risk of endometriosis. You may need a laparoscopy to definitively diagnose it and measure its severity. I think you'll find that this questionnaire will also help guide your discussion about fertility treatment. Enter the appropriate score after each question.

	No or Never (0)	Sometimes (1)	Yes or Always (2)
1. Do you have painful menstrual cycles?			
2. Do you experience pain during intercourse?			
3. Do you have bladder symptoms (frequent urination, burning on urination) during your menstrual cycles or have you been diagnosed with interstitial cystitis?			
4. Do you have bowel-related symptoms during your menstrual cycles or have you been diagnosed with IBS?			
5. Do you experience pain during bowel movements?			
6. Do you have a history of, or been previously diagnosed with, endometriosis?			
7. Did your mother or sister ever have endometriosis?			
8. Have you been pregnant within the last five years?			
9. Are you 35 years of age or older?			
10. Do you have naturally red hair?			

TOTAL: _____

Total your score. Here's the bottom line:

≤ 5: Your score does not rule out endometriosis, but suggests that your fertility treatment does not need to be delayed by diagnostic testing for this condition.

6–9: Discuss with your physician whether you should have a laparoscopy, especially if your symptoms are compromising your quality of life or if other useful information about your tubal health is needed.

≥ 10 (or if you answered yes to questions 2, 5, or 6): If you're having significant pain, I recommend you get a laparoscopy before deciding on your fertility treatment.

TWO DIAGNOSTIC TESTS TO SKIP

◆ **Cancer antigen 125 (CA125).** I discourage the use of this blood test. It measures the protein CA125, which is produced when the tissue covering the uterus, the ovaries, and other abdominal organs becomes irritated. The test was originally designed to track the growth of ovarian cancer, but CA125 also occurs at low levels in endometriosis, and, as it turns out, in many other disorders that affect the intestines and the liver. This leads to many "false positive" results, creating stress and anxiety without providing a clear diagnosis. It can, however, be used to track your response to treatment—falling levels suggest diminishing endometriosis, while rising levels suggest worsening endometriosis

◆ **Ultrasound.** Some tests create more questions than answers—an ultrasound used to assess endometriosis is one of them. An ultrasound can find signs suggestive of endometriosis, but it can't make a clear diagnosis and often mistakes other harmless clusters of cells for endometriosis. If you have this test for another reason and findings suggest endometriosis, your doctor may recommend a laparoscopy. I suggest that you disregard this ultrasound finding and base your decision upon your score on the "Endometriosis Risk Assessment" instead, to avoid an unnecessary and potentially expensive diagnostic surgery.

categorizes you as "minimal," "mild," "moderate," or "severe." These stages correspond to the factor levels 1 to 4 that I've created for other fertility factors and will help you decide which treatment path to take.

TREATING ENDOMETRIOSIS

Treatment of endometriosis should involve surgery to remove all possible lesions, but not everyone needs treatment. Your decision to treat should depend on the stage of your lesions as well as your symptoms. If you're having pain, no matter what stage you are, you deserve to feel better and should be treated. However, if your endometriosis is stage 3, but you're symptom free, you can proceed directly to IVF. Surgery is not considered a cure; after laparoscopy, 40 to 50 percent of women have a recurrence within five years. It's important to try to time your surgery three to six months before you'd like to conceive. Ironically, pregnancy has been shown to be the best treatment of endometriosis. Record your endometrial factor in the chart on page 226 to help determine what level treatment you may need to consider.

Case in Point

Kim and her husband Paul, both 28, came to see me after three years of trying to become pregnant and being diagnosed with "unexplained infertility." According to her medical record, Kim had suffered severe menstrual cramps for years, had a frequent need to urinate, and would often miss one or two days of work each month because of pelvic pain. To further add to her struggle, intercourse had become so painful that it was difficult to have sex each month around ovulation. I began by reassuring her that her "symptoms matter." That was important, since women with chronic pelvic pain are often told that they're imagining their discomfort or that it has psychological origins.

Kim's symptoms strongly suggested that she had both endometriosis and interstitial cystitis (IC). She said that her cycles had always been this way, as were her mother's, so she thought it was normal. I told her that endometriosis might be her primary obstacle to conception. I suggested we do a laparoscopy, which could also confirm that her fallopian tubes were unobstructed. I also explained I could treat the endometriosis to reduce her symptoms and improve her pregnancy rate. I gave her dietary recommendations to reduce her bladder symptoms.

I saw Kim and Paul about three weeks after her surgery, and she reported that her pain had improved. Then we sat down to review the surgical findings. I showed them photographs of the endometriosis lesions that were on her uterus and her left ovary. I also told them both tubes were open. Then, using staging sheets, I explained that the size and location of her lesions prior to surgery classified her problem as stage 2, but since I treated it during surgery, it should not impair her chance of pregnancy for the next several months to years.

I encouraged her to use the OV-Watch to monitor her fertile window. Kim also reported that since the surgery, she had less discomfort during sex. About six weeks later, I received an e-mail from Kim that she was pregnant. She said her bladder symptoms had disappeared and her pain was gone. She delivered a healthy girl.

Stage 1: Minimal

If you had very few superficial lesions of endometriosis, your surgeon probably removed them during your laparoscopy. This will improve your success rate slightly. If, for some reason, your lesions were not removed, I would *not* recommend having a second surgery to treat them.

AVOID MEDICAL TREATMENTS

You may be offered medical treatment with BioLimited hormones like Lupron or Zoladex. These injectable medications will suppress estrogen and interfere with ovulation, delaying your ability to conceive. They will also cause menopause-like symptoms. I don't recommend this for any woman who wants to get pregnant in the near future.

The additional expense and time are generally not justified. If you're not having symptoms, you can move forward with fertility treatment.

Stage 2: Mild

Most women with endometriosis fall into this group. The lesions are typically treated with laparoscopy, after which you're ready for your fertility treatment. Despite their popularity, lasers do not offer any improvement in outcome and may add additional cost to your surgery. Your doctor may offer you postoperative medication, like the BioLimited hormones Lupron or Zoladex, but as these suppress FSH and LH, which in turn suppresses ovulation, I do not recommend these medications if you'd like to become pregnant. They can also cause menopause-like symptoms.

Stage 3: Moderate

Some women develop advanced disease fairly quickly. Try to find a board-certified reproductive endocrinologist to perform the delicate surgery requiring the extensive removal of tissue in and around your reproductive organs. A specialist is also more likely to take steps to reduce injury to your ovaries and fallopian tubes, as well as avoid removal of sections of your ovary or do anything else that would compromise your ovarian reserve and your fertility. This procedure may be done via laparoscopy, but your surgeon may instead recommend a more traditional incision depending on the location and severity of your lesions.

Stage 4: Severe

Chances are your endometriosis has been a major health burden for you. In addition to causing fertility problems, it has probably been causing pain as well as problems with your digestive tract. Because of the extent of your disease, you are more likely to need surgery through an abdominal incision. Your doctor may recommend that a second surgeon be present to assist with treating any endometriosis on your colon or bladder. Your surgery should not only improve your quality of life, but will also provide a major improvement in your response to fertility treatment.

AN HERBAL REMEDY FOR ENDOMETRIOSIS

Many women with endometriosis continue to have pelvic pain even after surgical removal of all their lesions. In order to provide relief, many health care providers have used hormone-suppressing agents (BioLimited hormones or BioAntagonists) like Lupron or Zoladex. However these have not been shown to improve pregnancy rates and can delay your ability to become pregnant. Recently a third option has been investigated: pine bark extract.

A certain type of pine tree is known to have bark that contains a potent antioxidant/anti-inflammatory called *polyphenols.* In 2007, a large study randomly assigned women with endometriosis to take either a 30 mg capsule twice a day of a pine bark extract or to take Lupron. In only four weeks, all women experienced a reduction in their symptoms. Women using the herbal extract reported that pain was reduced by about 80 percent and cramping about 75 percent, which were about the same as those on Lupron. But the women on the extract continued to have regular menstrual cycles, whereas those on Lupron didn't, and those on the extract did not experience the menopausal side effects of Lupron. What's more, at least five women on the pine bark extract became pregnant. Finally, women on Lupron had a rebound return of symptoms when they went off the drug, whereas pine bark had no such effect. Talk to your doctor about whether you should consider taking this herbal remedy if you're in pain.

RECURRENT MISCARRIAGES

Experiencing the loss of a pregnancy can be exceedingly distressing, but having to go through it again and again is beyond devastating. About 5 percent of all couples experience three or more consecutive miscarriages, the official definition of *recurrent miscarriage.* But many other couples have one or two early pregnancy losses. A growing number of fertility specialists, myself included, are shunning the classical definition and treating people with two consecutive miscarriages or a total of

Case in Point

Katie was one of the most distraught patients that I had ever met. At 31, she and her husband, Dave, had suffered five miscarriages in seven years. They had been put through extensive testing, but I felt that they had been led astray. The evaluation had ruled out many potential factors that can contribute to recurrent miscarriage—uterine factor, blood-clotting disorders, genetic anomalies, and immunological factors—but did not find any possible causes for the miscarriages.

I immediately recognized that she had mild PCOS, based upon her acne, her weight, and the results of a prior ultrasound of her ovaries. Because she had regular menstrual cycles and did not have difficulty getting pregnant, PCOS was probably missed by her other doctors. But at five feet four inches, Katie weighed 206 pounds and had likely suffered from insulin resistance for several years, contributing to her progressive weight gain. I suggested that she wait at least three months while she tried to restore hormone balance and lose weight to further boost her success rate.

I started Katie on metformin to improve her insulin resistance as well as the oral contraceptive Yaz to help normalize her testosterone level. She began the Perfect Balance program, paying particular attention to boosting her fiber and switching to organic products. Over the next three months, she lost 20 pounds, and by six months her weight was down to 170 pounds—the lowest it had been in a decade. At that point, they were ready to try to conceive. She started doing yoga and was taking a prenatal vitamin; Dave was taking ConceptionXR to help optimize his sperm production.

Within two months of carefully timed intercourse, using the OV-Watch to monitor her fertile window, Katie was pregnant. Her progesterone level was low, so I placed her on Prometrium twice a day, and recommended she take a low-dose aspirin to minimize her risk of blood clotting, although this had not been a problem thus far. She followed up every two weeks, and we quietly celebrated each landmark—the appearance of the heartbeat, the first fetal movement, and the eight-week milestone she had never passed. At the end of her first trimester, I stopped the Prometrium but continued the metformin and the aspirin. She delivered a healthy baby girl.

three (a couple may have had a normal pregnancy between miscarriages). I and others find it hard to tell couples who have had two miscarriages to come back to see me after the third pregnancy loss, though many couples are actually told this.

Well over 50 percent of miscarriages occur within the first six weeks of pregnancy. After that, the miscarriage rate drops to about 10 percent. This strongly suggests that events surrounding implantation are the most critical to a successful pregnancy. Implantation requires a complex interaction of the embryo's genes, the woman's immune system, a healthy uterine environment, a good blood supply, and, most important, hormone balance. In two-thirds of all cases evaluated, more than one factor contributes to the problem. But with close monitoring, the chances of a successful pregnancy can be greatly improved.

Because there are so many contributing factors, you may be offered a variety of tests and treatments. I've sorted through those that are helpful and those that should be avoided because of their high cost and lack of proven effectiveness. In addition, some fertility treatments can actually do harm by increasing the chances of a miscarriage. Review this section carefully before you become pregnant, and consider reviewing it as soon as you have a positive pregnancy test.

No doctor has the ability to predict which pregnancy will miscarry and which one won't. In order to counsel couples more effectively, we look for risk factors to determine who needs additional testing and treatment. To help you gauge your own level of risk, take the following questionnaire, based on the most widely recognized risk factors.

RECURRENT MISCARRIAGE RISK ASSESSMENT

Answer the following questions.

1. Have you had three or more consecutive miscarriages?   Yes   No
2. Have you been pregnant within the last six months?   Yes   No
3. Do you have a blood-clotting disorder?   Yes   No
4. Was your labor pain-free (indicating an incompetent cervix) or unusually fast?   Yes   No
5. Do you have an autoimmune disorder like lupus or antiphospholipid antibody syndrome?   Yes   No
6. Do you have uterine factor 3 or 4?   Yes   No
7. Are you over 40 years of age or is your partner over 45?   Yes   No
8. Do you or you partner work around hazardous or toxic materials or chemicals?   Yes   No
9. Have you had a biopsy of the cervix—either a LEEP procedure or conization within the last six months?   Yes   No
10. Do you or your partner have a family history of recurrent miscarriage or infertility?   Yes   No

Total your score. Here's the bottom line:

If you answered yes to any three questions, or to question 1, 4, 5, 6, or 9, discuss your risk of miscarriage and the following measures with a fertility specialist. By planning ahead, you can take precautions to lower your risk and improve your outcome.

PREVENTING MISCARRIAGE

CONSIDER GENETIC TESTING. The vast majority of miscarriages occur in the first trimester, and at least half of these are caused by a chromosomal abnormality. This is by far the most common cause of miscarriage. As your chromosomes match up with your partners, errors can occur, and most of these errors lead to miscarriage.

The earlier your miscarriage occurred, the more likely it was caused by a genetic problem. For instance, studies on so-called *chemical pregnancies*—those that occur after a positive pregnancy test but before a pregnancy can be seen on an ultrasound—have shown that 70 percent are related to chromosomal anomalies. The incidence drops to about 50 percent during the rest of the first trimester and then to about 5 percent for those miscarriages that occur in the second or third trimester. The best way to confirm if your pregnancy loss was due to a chromosomal anomaly is to request a genetic analysis of the pregnancy tissue collected at the time of a D & C, the procedure used to remove any tissue that remains after a miscarriage. This is a valuable test that can help prevent future miscarriages, but, unfortunately, most doctors do not routinely do it, so you'll have to request it prior to your D & C. If the test shows that you had a *numeric chromosomal abnormality*—having one more chromosome than 46 or one less—this is a reassuring finding, since these abnormalities are considered random events and do not increase your risk of future miscarriages.

Ask Dr. Greene

Q Will taking steps to reduce a miscarriage increase my risk of having a child with a genetic abnormality?

A A common concern expressed by many patients is that intervening with nature by trying to reduce the chance of a miscarriage may increase the chance of delivering a child with an abnormality. That couldn't be further from the truth. If your miscarriage is due to a genetic factor, the supportive treatments I recommend will not be able to prevent the miscarriage. If, however, the reason for your previous miscarriages were hormonal imbalance, a blood-clotting problem, or an immune disorder, then treating this problem will not only reduce the chance of another miscarriage, but also *improve* your child's health.

For couples that have already experienced three or more miscarriages, there is a 3 percent risk of a different type of subtle chromosomal problem. There may be a missing piece of a chromosome, a damaged section, or, most commonly, a shuffling of the order of chromosomes (called a *translocation*). About 90 percent of all chromosomal problems are traced to the egg, suggesting that abnormal sperm typically don't function well enough to fertilize an egg. As you age, you have a greater risk of these subtle DNA problems. If you're not currently pregnant and have had three or more miscarriages, talk to your fertility specialist about whether a consultation with a geneticist may be useful for counseling and testing. If you are currently pregnant and you've had three miscarriages, or if you've had two and you're at least 38 years old, consider early genetic testing like *chorionic villus sampling (CVS)*, which is done four to five weeks earlier than an amniocentesis, to get information as early as possible on the health of your pregnancy.

RULE OUT UTERINE ANOMALIES. In 3 to 5 percent of couples that experience recurrent miscarriage, anatomical problems are a primary cause. I've discussed these in detail in chapter 11. Treating uterine factors can markedly reduce your risk of miscarriage.

LIMIT TESTING FOR IMMUNOLOGIC FACTORS. Many doctors recommend a barrage of immunologic tests, although these factors are among the least common causes of early pregnancy loss. Instead, by targeting a few key tests, which I describe below, you can feel reassured that this factor has been covered. But first a little background on how your immune system functions.

The white blood cells that make up your immune system react to *antigens*—proteins and other large molecules that are capable of causing an immune response. Some white blood cells attack antigens by producing *antibodies,* proteins that are tailor-made to attack a specific target. White blood cells can also create chemicals that promote *inflammation*—a reaction designed to attract more ominous white blood cells, called *natural killer (NK) cells,* which then identify and destroy foreign invaders. In the absence of inflammation, NK cells would otherwise pass by without noticing. Either antibodies or inflammatory reactions can precipitate a miscarriage.

First, let's consider the antibody response. Normally, we do not develop antibodies to our own antigens. If you do, you have an *autoimmune disorder* like lupus, rheumatoid arthritis, or multiple sclerosis. Women with autoimmune disorders are at an elevated risk of miscarriage. But other women may also have certain antibodies that put them at higher risk. The most common examples of these antibodies are those that can trigger abnormal blood clotting that can obstruct the blood supply to the developing baby. Here are the tests most commonly offered.

Antiphospholipid antibodies. Lipids (fats) that contain the mineral phosphorus (called *phospholipids*) are a normal component of the cell membranes and an essential part of the developing placenta. About 10 percent of women with infertility test positive for antibodies against these special lipids, raising their risk of forming blood clots. If you test positive, treatment with low-dose aspirin or heparin, which can prevent blood clots, may help your pregnancy progress normally. Talk to your fertility specialist about which treatment is most appropriate for you.

Antithyroid antibodies. If you test positive for antibodies against your own thyroid, an autoimmune condition called *Hashimoto's thyroiditis,* you may be at increased risk of a miscarriage. Some women with positive antibodies can develop hypothyroidism in response to the high estradiol levels that result from some fertility treatments. If your thyroid hormone is low, refer to my BioIdentical recommendations on page 232.

Antipaternal leukocyte antibody testing. Fertility specialists have debated the value of this test for years. Many years ago, studies began observing that late in the third trimester, some pregnant women developed antibodies to their partners' white blood cells, and it was assumed that they were exposed to these cells through their developing baby. Subsequently, researchers found that women with recurrent pregnancy loss were *less* likely to develop these antibodies. Even though we know that these antibodies are not needed to have a healthy pregnancy (not all women develop them), the idea emerged to treat a woman with recurrent miscarriage by exposing her to her partner's white blood cells so that she forms antibodies. Now we have enough research to conclude that this treatment does not improve pregnancy rates. Skip the test and the treatment.

The other type of immunologic disorder is an inflammatory reaction to antigens from your partner. The hormones (primarily progesterone) you produce early in pregnancy have an *immunomodulatory effect,* meaning that they suppress the white blood cells just enough so that the immune cells ignore antigens produced by your developing baby—the ones that were inherited from your partner. When the white blood cells don't abide by this diminished role, they may contribute to miscarriage. Around 1999, however, studies found that some popular treatments were ineffective, yet some doctors still test for and try to treat these conditions today.

Active immunization. This treatment entailed exposing women to their partner's white blood cells before conception to provoke their immune system to form antibodies. It was replaced by another equally ineffective treatment called *passive immunization,* in which women were given the actual antibodies from donors in the form of intravenous immunoglobulin (IVIG). You may still be offered these tests and treatments, but they are not recommended by the ASRM.

Natural killer cell disorder. The most abundant cells in the uterus prior to implantation are NK cells. Studies of women with recurrent miscarriage suggest that these cells are present in excess numbers,

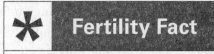

✳ Fertility Fact

Embryo Glue

It's estimated that only about half of all embryos that arrive in the uterus are able to implant. We now understand that a number of proteins on the embryo attach themselves to the endometrium before the embryo firmly implants itself. There is evidence that some IVF failures may be due to a failure of the embryo to bind to the uterine wall long enough for implantation to progress. This problem may be overcome simply by using particular types of culture media during subsequent cycles that would essentially coat the embryo with these sticky proteins, allowing it to "glue" itself to the endometrium until it implants. Although most patients don't need this experimental embryo glue, if you've experienced one or more failed IVF cycles, talk to your doctor about whether you'd benefit from it and if it's available.

probably due to chronic inflammation. The theory is that NK cells may be waiting in ambush for the embryo when it drops from the fallopian tube into the uterus. Some fertility centers offer cortisol to reduce the aggressiveness of NK cells, but this immune-suppression treatment is considered experimental. If your doctor recommends it, ask about any new research that supports his recommendation.

PREVENT BLOOD-CLOTTING DISORDERS. Implantation involves a delicate balance of about 20 proteins that affect the blood supply to the developing baby. First, these proteins promote the formation of blood vessels to support the pregnancy; then they promote some degree of blood clotting to reduce bleeding; and finally they dissolve blood clots when they form inappropriately. The process, however, can go awry during the rapid changes associated with early pregnancy. When the balance of proteins is tipped toward promoting clotting, it can cause placental blood vessels to become blocked, causing a miscarriage. There are several other blood-clotting conditions you might want to be tested for in order to reduce your chances of having another miscarriage. I describe two of the most common disorders below.

Hyperhomocysteinemia. When elevated, homocysteine can promote blood clotting. If your homocysteine is high, it may mean that you're not getting enough of the vitamin folic acid, which can increase the risk of your child being born with certain birth defects like spina bifida. Those with high homocysteine may need more than 400 mcg—the amount typically contained in prenatal vitamins. The test for homocysteine should be done when fasting, since certain foods can cause a false elevation.

Factor V Leiden deficiency. The most common inherited blood-clotting disorder is a birth defect involving a mutation in the protein called *factor V Leiden* that normally slows down blood clotting. Ask your doctor whether you should be tested for this or any of the other less-common blood-clotting disorder, based upon your medical and family history. If so, these can be treated with heparin in order to improve your chances of a successful pregnancy.

TAKE LOW-DOSE ASPIRIN. Taking an 81 mg dose of aspirin has been shown to help reduce recurrent miscarriage; aspirin thins the blood, reducing the risk of clotting, and it also reduces inflammation, lowering the chance that NK cells are activated.

MAINTAIN GOOD NUTRITION. Being very overweight or underweight is a risk for recurrent miscarriage. If your weight does not fall within the Perfect Balance Fertility Zone (having a body mass index between 19 and 25), review chapter 4 for tips on how to work toward a healthier weight. If you have recurrent miscarriage, pay particular attention to these dietary recommendations.

Eat a low-fat diet. A high-fat diet promotes inflammation, which can exacerbate immunological factors.

Take an omega-3 fatty acid supplement. This healthy fat can help improve blood flow to the placenta during implantation and lower the risk of blood-clot formation. I recommend the supplement Expecta LIPIL.

Avoid excess calories. If you're overeating, you may be increasing your levels of damaging free radicals. Recall that oxygen is needed to break down food, but as the oxygen is metabolized, it creates free radicals. The more you overeat, the more free radicals you form. Early embryo development occurs in a very low oxygen environment to reduce the risk of free radical formation during this vulnerable period. Some studies suggest that antioxidants like vitamin C and E may help reduce the miscarriage rate; however, lowering free radical formation by eating less and choosing fewer calorie-dense foods is even more effective.

Boost selenium. Low selenium levels have been observed in women with first trimester miscarriage. This mineral is an integral antioxidant that embryos rely on to protect their DNA. You need about 60 mcg of selenium per day. Walnuts are a good source, but you can get all the selenium that you need by eating a few Brazil nuts several times a week.

Go organic. Your developing fetus is susceptible to low levels of toxins that are considered within the acceptable range by current food production standards. This is one more compelling reason to choose organic foods when they're available.

CORRECT HORMONAL IMBALANCES. This is the most treatable factor contributing to miscarriage. The key hormones essential for establishing a healthy pregnancy are progesterone, thyroxine, and insulin.

Ask Dr. Greene

Q Can I use progesterone cream when I become pregnant?

A No, I recommend against it. I've been amazed by the growing popularity of progesterone creams to treat everything from PMS to hot flashes. Progesterone is very poorly absorbed through the skin, so I don't trust that it will provide the levels needed to ensure proper implantation. Moreover, at least one recent study found that women with recurrent miscarriage are at high risk of developing skin irritation when progesterone is applied topically. Women have reported severe skin irritation after a progesterone injection as well. I recommend the use of progesterone from an FDA-approved source that can be consistently absorbed and is not associated with skin reactions, such as the Prometrium pill, the vaginal gels Crinone or Prochieve, or the vaginal tablet Endometrin.

Progesterone. It has long been debated whether low progesterone causes miscarriage, leading some doctors to prescribe progesterone and others not to when their newly pregnant patients have low progesterone. At last, the jury is in. As you may recall, when an egg is released, it leaves behind the corpus luteum, which produces progesterone. Several recent studies have confirmed that *luteal insufficiency,* or the inability of the corpus luteum to produce enough progesterone, is a common contributing cause of early miscarriage. As women reach their later reproductive years, their ovaries often become less effective at making progesterone. In addition, studies suggest that some of the ovulation-inducing hormones used in fertility treatments can trigger an imbalance between estradiol and progesterone that contributes to luteal insufficiency. Recall that progesterone tempers estradiol's growth-promoting effects on endometrial cells, allowing the endometrium to mature and prepare for implantation. I recommend having your blood level checked about a week after ovulation. If your progesterone is below 20 ng/ml, request a prescription for BioIdentical Prometrium (a pill), the vaginal gel Crinone or Prochieve, or the vaginal tablet Endometrin. Discuss with your doctor what dose is most appropriate based on your results.

Dr. Greene

> If you are thyroid deficient and require a daily dose of thyroid replacement hormone, I recommend that you talk to your doctor about increasing your dose by two extra pills per week as soon as you've had a positive pregnancy test. You can space them out so that the extra tablets are separated by three or four days.

Insulin. Women with diabetes are about two to three times more likely to have a miscarriage or a child with a developmental problem. Many studies show that women with PCOS, which is associated with insulin resistance, are also at high risk for early pregnancy loss. Insulin plays an important role in establishing the metabolic rate of the endometrium and, in so doing, supports implantation. But at high levels, it can interfere with implantation by boosting testosterone. Numerous studies have shown that taking the insulin-sensitizing drug metformin reduces miscarriage rates and birth defects in women with insulin resistance. It is classified as pregnancy category B—meaning that thousands of women have taken this during pregnancy without any increase in the incidence of birth defects. Talk to your fertility specialist to see if this would be an appropriate therapy for you, and refer to chapter 13 for more information on metformin.

Thyroxine. A severe imbalance of the thyroid hormone, thyroxine, is clearly associated with pregnancy loss, but whether mild thyroid deficiencies also contribute to miscarriage is still a matter of debate. I believe even a mild deficiency can contribute based on the fact that the hormone HCG, which is released early in pregnancy, triggers the release of thyroxine, suggesting that thyroid hormone may play some role in implantation.

If you have low thyroid function based upon a blood test performed when you're not pregnant, you should repeat the test shortly after you've conceived. If it remains low, ask your fertility specialist to consider giving you a low-dose BioIdentical supplement of thyroxine, about 25 to 50 mcg/day. It may help prevent a miscarriage, and because it's a very low dose, it, shouldn't cause symptoms of *hyper*thyroidism (like rapid heart rate or anxiety) for the vast majority of patients.

◆　◆　◆

Congratulations. You have arrived at the moment when you have enough information to decide on your treatment. In the introduction to the treatment section, I'll help you determine which treatment is best for you, based on your individual factors.

4

Your Fertility Plan: Making It Happen

Introduction: Fertility Treatments

After months, if not years, of having negative pregnancy tests, many couples feel a sense of renewed hope when they embark on treating their infertility. The first visit to a specialist can relieve some depressed feelings, but it can also create some anxiety about what's to come. If you have followed my step-by-step program, you will not only have a healthier hormone profile, but you should also have everything you need to make the best decisions about your fertility treatment. It will still be a challenge, as the sheer number of options available and their subtle differences can be downright confusing. I know that it's easier to let a physician direct your treatment, but the risks of not being an equal partner are unnecessary tests, inappropriate treatment, and wasted time, emotions, and money.

I hope that I have helped you define your fertility factors and your needs. The chart you have been filling out on page 226 as you progressed through the diagnostic section will direct you to which chapter in this section you'll find the most appropriate treatment for you: the basic reproductive treatments in chapter 13 or the advanced reproductive techniques in chapter 14. Within each chapter, when appropriate, I'll specifically recommend certain treatments based on your fertility factors. I suggest you read both chapters as some of the basic treatments are components of the advanced techniques. It's also helpful to have a broad perspective of what's available before you and your partner decide what treatment will be right for you. In either case, keep in mind that restoring and maintaining hormone balance are going to be key elements in your success, no matter what path you take.

One observation I've made over the years is that most couples have waited so long to see a fertility specialist that when they finally do, they feel somewhat desperate and want the most aggressive treatment strategies. Some fertility centers are more than willing to oblige, as these are also the biggest moneymakers for them. It's up to you to resist this urge and start with treatments that are most appropriate.

ESTIMATING YOUR TREATMENT NEEDS

In order to help you and your partner apply what you've learned about your own situation, I've developed the Perfect Balance Fertility Nomogram for you to estimate your treatment needs based on your fertility factors. I've based this nomogram on my years of experience treating fertility patients. This is an estimate of where you should consider beginning this next leg of your journey. You'll need to take this information and discuss it with your health care provider. If she does not agree, you need to listen to her explanations. It's possible that a newer treatment or test may have been developed or shown to be effective for you since the final editing of this book. It's also possible that there is something that is unique to you and your partner that I haven't covered in this book. Nonetheless, this should give you a solid starting point for beginning your discussion of your treatment.

FINDING THE RIGHT SPECIALIST FOR YOUR NEEDS

As more and more doctors claim that they treat infertility, it's important for you to be able to distinguish who is qualified to treat you. Some well-intended clinicians will only offer you the most advanced treatment that they are capable of performing. But it may be more than you need. Others may not even be able to provide the level of services that you require. Yet they may not have the knowledge or integrity to refer you to someone that does. That's why you have to be a savvy patient. For guidance on what type of specialist is most qualified to treat you, go to Appendix C.

Perfect Balance Fertility Nomogram

Using your fertility factors from the chart on page 226, draw separate straight lines connecting each female factor to the male factor (or the need for a sperm donor). Each line will intersect the heavy shaded line, which represents the continuum of treatment, with basic treatments at one end and advanced treatments at the other. Whichever point of inter- section is farthest right on the shaded line indicates my best estimate of your beginning level of treatment—basic or advanced. If your lines intersect on the left side of the centerline, you can focus your efforts on the basic treatments I will describe in chapter 13. If your point of intersection is to the right of center, you can go directly to the advanced treatment options I describe in chapter 14. Throughout the next two chapters, I'll provide even more specific guidance based on your individual factors.

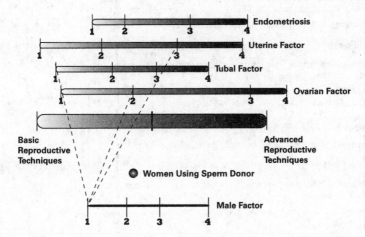

The dotted lines represent the fertility factors of one couple, Sheila and Peter. Sheila has uterine factor 3, ovarian factor 2 (and tubal factor 1—minimal), and Peter has male factor 1 (also minimal). The line farthest to the right falls to the left of center on the treatment continuum, suggesting that the couple begin with basic fertility treatment.

By understanding what treatment options are appropriate for you and your partner, you can direct the discussion with your doctor toward those that you're most comfortable with as a starting place. Then it's a process of listening and negotiating. If you feel your doctor does not appreciate your thorough forethought on your fertility, consider seeking a specialist that will. You deserve that respect.

YOUR FERTILITY FACTORS

Record your factors in this chart. After the chart is complete, refer to the nomogram on page 225 to estimate the level of treatment that you should consider.

Male Factor	Your Factor Level
MF1 (presumed fertile). You have a normal semen analysis.	
MF2 (mild). You have minor changes in your semen and may benefit from treatment.	(Example: MF2)
MF3 (moderate). Your semen count is having a major impact on your fertility.	
MF4 (severe). You have severe male factor infertility and will need ART or a sperm donor in order to conceive.	

Ovarian Factor	Your Factor Level
OF1 (presumed fertile). Your ovarian health should not factor into your fertility options.	
OF2 (mild). Your ovaries are mildly impacting your ability to conceive.	
OF3 (moderate). The quality of your follicles is a significant factor in your ability to conceive.	
OF4 (severe). Your ovaries are a major obstacle to your infertility.	

Tubal Factor	Your Factor Level
TF1 (presumed fertile). There's no evidence that you have any tubal factor limiting your fertility.	
TF2 (mild). Your tubal factor doesn't limit your options, but it should raise your awareness of your tubal health.	
TF3 (moderate). You have significant tubal factor; your options depend on the specific damage to your tubes and its cause.	
TF4 (severe). Your tubal factor severely limits your options.	

Uterine Factor	Your Factor Level
UF1 (presumed fertile). Your uterine factor should not impact your treatment choices.	
UF2 (mild). A minor problem has been identified based upon your test results.	
UF3 (moderate). You have a significant anatomical malformation that is moderately impacting your fertility; your options depend on the specific cause.	
UF4 (severe). Your uterine factor can't be resolved or corrected; discuss your options with your fertility specialist.	

Endometriosis Staging	Your Factor Level
Leave this blank if you have never had endometriosis.	
EF1 (minimal). You had minimal superficial lesions either removed by your surgeon or not removed, but it should not affect your treatment.	
EF2 (mild). You had mild lesions treated by laparoscopy. You're free to choose any treatment.	
EF3 (moderate). You had moderate lesions around your reproductive organs that were treated before pursuing fertility treatment.	
EF4 (severe). You had severe lesions around your reproductive and abdominal organs that need to be treated before attempting fertility treatment.	

13 Basic Reproductive Treatment

For most couples with infertility, their key to success lies in basic fertility treatments like those that promote hormone balance and therapies that promote the development of eggs and support the production of healthy sperm, rather than in advanced reproductive techniques like IVF. These treatments may require some patience, but the amount of money saved through these less-expensive therapies makes them appealing to many. They also tend to come with lower risks of multiple births and other pregnancy complications if managed correctly. I'll review the simplest therapies that restore hormone balance and progress to those that promote egg development, fertilization, and implantation.

Basic fertility options are available through any reproductive endocrinologist. Some of these treatments are also available through more highly trained ob-gyns who have stayed up to date on advancements in the diagnosis and treatment of fertility problems (they should be members of ASRM; see www.asrm.org). A general care provider who understands how various hormonal imbalances can interfere with your fertility may be able to administer and monitor the treatments that focus on correcting hormonal imbalances (refer to Appendix C).

SUCCESS RATES

One question I'm always asked about a treatment is "What is its success rate?" It's a difficult question to answer. Often the success statistics are misleading because they vary widely among clinics and even vary within the same clinic, depending on a couple's individual fertility factors. In addition, each success rate reported is only as good as the physician and the appropriateness of the treatment provided. I try to put success rates in perspective for my patients, based on their fertility factors and my own success with the procedures they're considering. I also think it's easy for couples to get confused by general percentages. For example, if a given procedure has a predicted success rate of 30 percent, that means it is 30 percent for each attempt, not that their chance will rise to 60 percent or 90 percent if they try it a second and third time. I recommend that you talk to your fertility specialist about what your predicted monthly pregnancy rate is without treatment (based upon your fertility factors) compared to what it would be with treatment. Then ask how couples with a comparable set of circumstances have responded at their center to each treatment you're considering. This specific information will give you a realistic reading of your chance of success.

HORMONE-BALANCING THERAPIES

If you have any of the imbalances in this section, treatment will improve your chance of ovulation and reduce your risk of miscarriage. If your partner has an imbalance, correcting it will boost the quality and quantify of his sperm. If you choose to treat these imbalances, you will definitely improve your chance of becoming pregnant. However, if you do go on to additional treatment like ovarian stimulation with intrauterine insemination or even to ART, correcting the following key hormonal imbalances first will improve your success and your health.

Insulin Resistance

If you are obese or have PCOS, you probably have insulin resistance and high insulin levels. This may be your greatest obstacle to pregnancy. Having high insulin is a known cause of infertility, and contributes to miscarriage. Because of this hormone imbalance, when women with PCOS become pregnant, they're at a higher risk of gestational diabetes,

ACUPUNCTURE TO BALANCE HORMONES

Acupuncture has recently been recommended as a treatment for infertility. Some research suggests that it may be able to increase ovulation rates in some women with PCOS, though the data is inconsistent. It does appear to reduce anxiety and depression in women experiencing an increase in stress hormones related to their infertility. Discuss this option with your fertility specialist, and if you choose to use acupuncture, avoid the use of Chinese herbs, which may interfere with the medications used to treat infertility.

excessive weight gain, pregnancy-induced hypertension, preeclampsia, preterm delivery, and the need for a cesarean section due to a large baby. To treat insulin resistance, it's best to use an insulin-sensitizing drug, and though there are several to choose from, I prefer metformin, available as a generic or the brand name Glucophage, Fortamet, or Glumetza. It is among the most effective, safest, and least expensive treatments available. This oral medication works by making your liver more sensitive to insulin, allowing it to take up more glucose from the bloodstream. The liver then stores it as glycogen and releases it when blood sugar is low between meals and while you're sleeping. By helping

BEWARE OF OUTDATED SURGERY TO CORRECT HORMONE IMBALANCE

In the past, the cysts associated with PCOS were thought to be a barrier to fertility because they generate hormones that inhibit egg development. To lower levels of these unhelpful hormones, surgeons used to remove a wedge-shaped piece of the ovary, along with its cysts. Unfortunately, the correction was only temporary, and scar tissue would often create a new fertility obstacle. A later adaptation was the "Wiffle-ball procedure," in which a laser was used to drill 15 to 20 small holes in each ovary to drain the cysts. This would temporarily restore ovulation and did reduce scar tissue formation. Both of these expensive treatments, however, do reduce ovarian reserve, since some healthy, dormant eggs are damaged in the process. I do not recommend surgical therapy for correcting this hormonal imbalance.

remove sugar from the blood, metformin lowers your body's need to produce extra insulin. Based on more than a dozen studies, metformin will increase your rate of ovulation by about four times. Nearly one in every three women with irregular menstrual cycles and insulin resistance will begin ovulating on this treatment alone. If there are no other factors contributing to infertility, about half of those that begin ovulating will conceive within six months if they're also using an ovulation monitor. Lowering insulin can also boost progesterone production, reduce the chance of blood clotting, and normalize your immune response, reducing the chance of miscarriage.

If you're trying to lose weight, studies show that combining metformin with dietary and lifestyle changes like those in the Perfect Balance program will help you lose weight twice as fast as by either diet or medication alone. What's more, you'll lose abdominal weight that contributes to insulin resistance.

Some doctors aren't aware of metformin's safety record, and may advise you to avoid it. Metformin is a pregnancy category B drug—meaning that over the last several decades, there has been no evidence that it can increase the risk of birth defects. In 2001, the ASRM published a position paper supporting the use of insulin-sensitizing drugs in women trying to conceive, citing their strong safety and effectiveness records. For treating women with PCOS or obesity combined with infertility, the typical dose ranges from 1500 to 2000 mg a day.

Ask Dr. Greene

Q I've heard that metformin can have side effects. What if I can't tolerate them?

A The only common side effect of metformin is an upset stomach, occurring in about 15 percent of people. To prevent side effects, try these strategies. First, begin with a low dose, about 500 mg each day, and take it with dinner to slow absorption. Over two to three weeks, gradually increase the dose until you reach the recommended 1,500 to 2,000 mg a day. You might want to consider the extended-release formula, which tends to be better tolerated. My patients tolerate Glumetza the best. If that doesn't work, talk to your doctor about one of the alternative insulin-sensitizing agents like Actos. Although this hasn't been as well studied and won't help you lose weight, it rarely causes upset stomach and can still be used to effectively restore hormone balance.

TREAT HIGH PROLACTIN

An estimated 17 percent of women with infertility have high prolactin levels, which may inhibit ovulation. Men with sexual dysfunction also have a higher incidence of high prolactin levels. If you are diagnosed with high prolactin, it is important to restore this hormone to normal levels to improve your chance of conceiving. The two most popular medications for restoring hormone balance are Parlodel (taken daily) or Dostinex (taken twice weekly). These oral medications mimic the effects of dopamine, which suppresses the release of prolactin, but they don't cause the euphoria associated with dopamine release. If high prolactin is your only fertility factor, then this treatment alone is associated with a pregnancy rate of 60 to 80 percent within one year of initiating this treatment.

Thyroid

Maintaining a healthy balance of thyroid hormones is critical because of the role these hormones play in normal egg development, fertilization, and successful implantation. But it is especially important for the success of fertility treatment. If treatment like ovulation induction—when you're given hormones to stimulate the release of eggs—is initiated without correcting hypothyroidism (low thyroid hormone), studies show that eggs will often fail to fertilize. This is because ovulation induction, the primary fertility treatment used for women, causes rapid increases in estradiol, and as estradiol levels rise, the amount of active thyroid hormone or thyroxine (T4) in the blood naturally drops down. The health exams you take prior to beginning fertility treatment will typically detect hypothyroidism. If you're already on thyroid replacement, you'll need to increase your dose as estrogen rises throughout your treatment cycle. Your doctor should instruct you on when and how much to increase your dose.

If you have normal thyroid levels at the outset of treatment, your body will naturally boost the production of thyroxine when it senses the rise in estrogen. This is a great example of how your body adjusts hormones to maintain perfect hormone balance. But if you have borderline low-normal levels, talk to your doctor about simply starting a low dose of thyroid hormone when you start fertility treatment. Be forewarned that endocrinologists disagree on whether to treat borderline or *subclinical* hypothyroidism, but studies suggest that 1 to 4 percent of women with infertility have subclinical hypothyroidism contributing to their low pregnancy rate. In addition, low thyroid level can result in a child with a preventable learning disability. Given the risks, and that borderline low thyroid is easy to test for and inexpensive to treat, I recommend treating it. Currently, I usually treat it with BioIdentical thyroxine like Synthroid or Levothroid; the risk of treatment is minimal as well. If it has been more than one year since your last thyroid panel, ask your physician whether you should have your thyroid levels reevaluated.

OVULATION INDUCTION AND OVULATION ENHANCEMENT

The cornerstone of fertility treatment is the use of hormones to deliberately shift a woman's hormone balance to promote the maturation and release of fertile oocytes—a process referred to as *ovulation induction* or *ovulation enhancement* (falling under the umbrella acronym OI). Induction is used in women who are not ovulating and enhancement is used to increase the number of eggs in women who are ovulating to improve a couple's chance of an egg being fertilized and implanting. These treatments work by raising pregnancy-promoting hormones like FSH and LH. Many couples will become pregnant using only these medications, though several attempts may be necessary.

These hormone treatments do, however, create an increased risk of a pregnancy with a multiple gestation (e.g., twins, triplets, quadruplets, and quintuplets). Multiple gestations come with a markedly increased risk of preterm labor, low birth weight, preeclampsia, gestational diabetes, and postpartum hemorrhage. In order to reduce the

THE HORMONE PLAYERS

◆ **Estradiol** sends signals to the brain to help monitor egg development; when estradiol levels reach a certain threshold, they signal the brain to trigger ovulation.

◆ **Follicle-stimulating hormone (FSH)** recruits follicles and signals the ovaries to prepare a cohort of eggs to mature in preparation for ovulation.

◆ **Luteinizing hormone (LH).** Continuous low-level LH signals promote the production of estradiol by the ovary. A surge of LH is released by the brain each month to trigger ovulation.

ONE BABY AT A TIME

One of the major risks of fertility treatments is having multiple births. The rate of multiples, as a percentage of all pregnancies in the United States, has continued to rise since the modern era of fertility treatment began in 1980. But spurred by the ASRM's call to reverse the trend, fertility specialists have attempted to lower the incidence of triplet and higher-order pregnancies in couples undergoing more advanced treatments like IVF, largely by reducing the number of embryos they transfer back into a woman's uterus. Their efforts have reduced the proportion of triplets and higher-order pregnancies from 7 percent in 1996 to 3 percent in 2004. The rate of twins, though, has continued to rise as has the rate of multiple pregnancies associated with ovulation induction and ovulation enhancement. Much of this rise can be attributed to nonspecialists treating patients, and part of it can be blamed on overzealous treatment by specialists who are not carefully monitoring their patients. Though success rates and other details of IVF-type treatments are monitored by the CDC, basic fertility treatments are not, leaving providers accountable to no authority except their patients. Through your vigilance, you can reduce your own risk. Here are some common misconceptions about multiple births that you should consider as you move forward with your treatment.

◆ **Myth #1: Multiple pregnancies are *not* a risk.** About one in five couples report that they would prefer to have a twin pregnancy, according to patient surveys. This suggests a lack of awareness of the higher risks associated with multiples, including pregnancy complications and low-birth-weight babies. In addition, because of the risks to the fetuses of triplets or higher-order pregnancies, many couples are faced with the agonizing decision of whether they should have a reduction, essentially compromising one or more developing embryos to assure a safer birth and better health for the remaining two.

◆ **Myth #2: Only IVF increases your risk of multiples.** In fact, basic treatments are responsible for about 40 percent of multiple births. Talk to your provider about using ultrasound and blood tests to monitor your progress in order to avoid overstimulation of your ovaries during *any* treatment.

◆ **Myth #3: Seeing a fertility specialist (as opposed to your OB) increases your risk of multiples.** Any fertility treatment can increase your risk of having a multiple birth, but in general, a board-certified reproductive endocrinologist is the most qualified to keep your risk down to the lowest level possible. There is, however, great variation among physicians, whether they are specialists or not. Various studies suggest that when OI is combined with intrauterine insemination (placing the sperm directly into the uterus), multiple birth rates vary from 5 to 29 percent per couple. I believe this wide range reflects the level of care and skill of the physician. I can assure you from my own practice, which averages less than 5 percent twins and a very rare incidence of triplets (<0.05 percent) of all pregnancies, that the goal of reducing the odds of multiples is achievable.

Ask Dr. Greene

Q Does clomiphene increase my risk of developing cancer?

A No, but this is a common concern that was triggered by a very poorly designed study that was widely publicized several years ago. The investigators asked women with ovarian cancer if they had ever taken this drug. The problem is, it's likely that some of the subjects who took clomiphene for infertility never got pregnant. Never bearing a child raises any woman's risk of ovarian cancer, because pregnancy is protective against the disease. So it was never clear whether the increased risk detected in the study was due to the clomiphene or because the study group had an above average number of women who never bore children. Since then, studies have failed to confirm an increase in the risk when all risk factors were properly adjusted for.

risk of multiple gestations, yet improve the pregnancy rate, most fertility specialists will monitor their patient's response to OI hormones with ultrasound examinations, which measures the number of follicles that are growing and maturing adequately. Some also order blood tests to confirm the rise in estradiol—levels increase as more follicles mature. Yet there are physicians who will simply give a woman a prescription and an instruction sheet on how to check for ovulation and when to have intercourse and not monitor the effects of the hormones, which can lead to overstimulation of the ovaries. I feel this hands-off treatment is irresponsible, as it can lead to multiples as well as a dangerous condition called *ovarian hyperstimulation syndrome* (see page 237). It's also less effective.

Several medications are available for OI. Your decision, unfortunately, may be largely based on how much you can pay. There are some choices that are clearly much better than others, but they are exponentially pricier, and some options are not offered by every physician or fertility center. Here is a description of your options and a brief explanation of their pros and cons. I have listed the oral medications first because they tend to be less expensive, but they are also less potent and may come with more side effects. *My tips: All of the following OI therapies are a good starting point for couples with MF1 or MF2, and some couples with MF3, as well as women working with a donor sperm. They're also appropriate for women with OF1, OF2, TF1, or TF2, and some with TF3, UF1 to UF3, and EF1 and EF2.*

Clomid, Serophene (**BioLimited estradiol**). These medications (generic name: clomiphene), are the most widely used ovarian stimulation drugs. They block the estrogen receptors in the brain, much like an uncut key can occupy a door lock but is unable to open it. In doing so, they essentially block the estradiol produced by your ovaries from reaching your brain, giving your brain the false impression that your estradiol levels are low. In response, your brain releases extra FSH and LH, which both trigger the production of more estradiol and recruit additional follicles to mature in your

 Fertility Fact

Clomiphene Resistance

The results of many studies reveal that about 50 percent of women will ovulate on the 50 mg dose of clomiphene. By increasing the dose to 100 mg in those that don't respond initially, the ovulation rate rises to 75 percent. When combined with intrauterine insemination, successful ovulation induction with clomiphene yields a pregnancy rate of between 15 and 20 percent per cycle. Within four cycles, most patients that will conceive on clomiphene have done so. Yet about 25 percent of couples that were predicted to respond don't—a situation called *clomiphene resistance*.

Many women with PCOS are clomiphene resistant. For women who are overweight or obese, losing about 5 percent of their weight will often improve clomiphene responsiveness, as will taking metformin. If neither of these options is successful or appealing, the standard recommendation is to move on to a more-expensive treatment option.

I disagree with this approach and suggest that you consider a one-month course of an oral contraceptive instead. One study found that when clomiphene-resistant women were placed on birth control pills for one month, followed by a cycle of clomiphene at 100 mg, the ovulation rate was 71 percent. Of the women that repeated clomiphene without intervening with a birth control, only 8 percent ovulated, demonstrating that balancing hormones the month before improves the response of the follicles. Over half of the women that became responsive by using the birth control pill between clomiphene cycles were pregnant within six treatment cycles.

ovaries. Typically, you are placed on one 50 mg tablet per day for five days beginning on day 3 to 5 of your menstrual cycle. You should have an ultrasound on menstrual day 12—just before ovulation—to determine if your response to the medication was adequate. This should create two to four mature eggs. If not, the clomiphene is increased during the next cycle in order to get a more robust response. *Pros:* Clomiphene is inexpensive, costing about $40 to $50 a cycle, and is taken orally. *Cons:* A lot of women feel awful on it because it triggers symptoms similar to those of mild menopause, including hot flashes, mood changes, and sleeplessness. On rare occasions, it can induce temporary visual disturbances. Also, it's difficult to predict the correct dose for each woman, meaning that you may have to repeat the procedure several times before finding the dose that can stimulate your eggs. Some women, including most PCOS patients, won't respond to it at all. Finally, if you take it one day too late, it can block implantation. *My tips: Any of the injectable BioIdentical or BioSimilar hormones that I list below are better than clomiphene, but its affordable price makes it more appealing to many.*

> ## Did you know ?
>
> Taking a birth control pill for one month in between ovulation induction cycles can improve your success rate exponentially.

Femara (BioAntagonist estradiol). I currently do not recommend this drug because of safety concerns that have recently arisen. In 2006, the manufacturer of Femara issued a warning that this drug should not be used for OI because of a potentially elevated risk of birth defects. A larger study is looking into whether this was a real finding, but I recommend avoiding it until that issue has been fully investigated. Femara had become popular over the last several years as a way to lower the amount of estradiol produced by a woman's ovaries instead of blocking the receptors in her brain. As with clomiphene, your brain is tricked into releasing a larger amount of FSH. The typical dose is 2.5 to 5.0 mg per day (one or two tablets) for days 3 through 8 of a woman's cycle. *Pros:* Typically one to three mature oocytes develop. Femara has fewer side effects than clomiphene. Other research suggests that it may offer a similar pregnancy rate as clomiphene, but with a lower incidence of multiple pregnancies. *Cons:* It's currently not considered safe to take.

OVARIAN HYPERSTIMULATION SYNDROME

The most potentially serious complication of ovulation induction is *ovarian hyperstimulation syndrome (OHSS),* an exaggerated response by the ovaries to the hormonal manipulation. This occurs in about 3 percent of women receiving injectable therapies and appears to be triggered by the pregnancy hormone HCG (a replica of LH that's used to trigger ovulation). Following the injection, HCG levels rise but then subside unless a woman becomes pregnant, at which point she'll start producing more HCG. In some women, high HCG produces the hormone VEGF (vascular endothelial growth factor), which causes severe bloating, fluid retention, and an increased risk of blood clots. In the most severe cases, it can require hospitalization and even monitoring in the intensive care unit. Although this condition can't always be prevented, understanding your risk factors and careful monitoring of your response to OI drugs will dramatically reduce your chances of developing it and prevent it from progressing if it's detected early—in the first couple of weeks after you're given these medications.

Your symptoms matter! The earliest signs of OHSS are lower abdominal or pelvic discomfort, mild nausea, vomiting, and diarrhea. If you gain more than two pounds per day, notice an increase in your waist size, or you have a reduced amount of urine, you may be having a severe reaction, so notify your doctor immediately.

Your risk of developing OHSS is increased if you become pregnant and:

* You have PCOS.
* You're using high doses of injectable drugs to induce ovulation.
* Your estradiol level is high.
* You're less than 25 years old.
* You're below normal weight.
* You've had OHSS before.

Follistim, Gonal-F (BioIdentical FSH). This is my preferred treatment since it is formulated in a sterile laboratory and is identical to your natural FSH, making it the safest approach. Rather than tricking your brain, the BioIdentical FSH simply signals your ovaries to trigger more oocytes to mature. You and your partner are taught how to inject a premixed syringe with a very small needle at home. You will typically have daily injections just below the skin (subcutaneous) for seven to nine days. *Pros:* You won't waste a cycle using the wrong

TIMING IS EVERYTHING

On occasion, we find that the "fertile window" may occur during an inconvenient time. For instance, during a fertility treatment cycle for one couple I was treating, the male partner was called away as part of a crew fighting a large brushfire in another state. As the woman's ovaries were already responding to the Follistim, I lowered the dose to try to slow her response rather than abandon the cycle, since her husband was due home in a day or so. I suggested she use the BioAntagonist Antagon, which blocks the release of LH, to delay her ovulation. A couple of days later, her husband returned, so we triggered ovulation and proceeded with the intrauterine insemination as planned. They conceived and she delivered a healthy baby.

dose as you may on clomiphene because your response can be monitored with ultrasound (and the occasional blood test), and your doctor can adjust the dose or continue use of the drug until the ideal number of follicles have matured. *Cons:* This is a potent medication and you should only use it under the care of an experienced physician in order to minimize your risk of a multiple gestation and the very serious ovarian hyperstimulation syndrome (see sidebar on page 237). As with most injections, localized bruising, redness, pain, or itching at the injection site may occur. Unfortunately, this injectable therapy is exponentially more expensive than clomiphene, costing about $500 to $600 per cycle. *My tips: I often recommend a more conservative dosing schedule than some fertility specialists. I use mild ovarian stimulation to mature a few very high-quality oocytes that are more likely to fertilize and implant (based on their microscopic appearance), rather than mature a dozen less-fertile ones, as some other specialists do.*

Bravelle, Fertinex (BioSimilar FSH). These are purified forms of FSH that are extracted from the urine of menopausal women. The medication is injected once or twice each day in a similar fashion to the BioIdentical FSH, and also requires that you're monitored by ultrasound. The drug is continued for as long as it takes for the desired number of follicles to mature. *Pros:* It tends to be less expensive than BioIdentical FSH. *Cons:* It is packaged individually in vials that require you to mix and dilute the medication prior to injection. It's also slightly less potent than the BioIdentical formu-

Case in Point

When I first met Kristin, 28, and Stephen, 32, they were already frustrated. They had recently learned that the doctor who had been managing their treatment for more than a year was not a fertility specialist, as he had claimed. They were diagnosed with unexplained infertility, and had already gone through six courses of ovulation induction using clomiphene. None was successful.

After taking a thorough medical history, I explained that Kristin had PCOS. She was stunned that her previous health care provider had missed the diagnosis. I started her on metformin and the Perfect Balance program, and suggested that they should try to conceive on their own for six months while Kristin's ovaries responded to their new hormonal milieu. Kristin, understandably, was eager to proceed immediately with treatment, so I instructed them to call my office after her next menstrual cycle began. Our plan was to keep her on metformin and use Bioidentical FSH for ovulation induction. We also agreed to include intrauterine insemination (IUI).

They conceived on their very first treatment cycle, but in her fifth week, she miscarried. I placed Kristin on a birth control pill for several months to allow her body to fully recover. Although I tried to reassure her that their initial success was reason to be very optimistic about their prognosis, I could feel their growing despair. We tried two more cycles of OI/IUI, during which their frustration and stress began to rise again. Although I reminded them that Kristin had only been on the insulin-balancing program for a few months and would not experience the full benefits for at least three more months, they wanted to try a more intensive treatment, such as IVF. I felt strongly that they should wait and suggested they get a second opinion from another reproductive endocrinologist. Their second opinion confirmed Kristin's diagnosis of PCOS, and reassured them that the OI/IUI was appropriate. He acknowledged that IVF was a good option for them, but agreed that it was a bit premature to abandon the approach I had recommended. We proceeded as we had before. On the very next cycle, Kristin conceived. Following the Perfect Balance program for a bit longer may have been one of the most important things she did to conceive. Kristin continued the metformin to maintain hormone balance throughout the pregnancy. She delivered a healthy boy a few days after her due date.

our story

Robert: One reason I felt strongly that Kristin should try again with ovulation induction before proceeding to IVF was that I really identified with her experience. Even though our details were different, we seemed to be following the same path. When Kristin arrived at our practice as a new patient, Morgan had just had the miscarriage. Then Kristin conceived, but five weeks later she miscarried, too. The depth of Kristin's disappointment made me want to reveal what Morgan and I had gone through, but I couldn't because we had not told anyone about our own efforts to become pregnant. Just around the time that Kristin miscarried, Morgan and I had made the decision to move on to IVF. And just after our IVF cycle failed, Kristin started voicing her frustration with OI and wanted to try IVF. I really wanted to save them the expense and hassles of undergoing an unnecessary IVF cycle like we had, so I recommended a second opinion. When Kristin returned to our practice to resume her OI treatment, she conceived. A few months later, Morgan conceived, and both she and Kristin carried their pregnancies to term. Together, these pregnancies made me even more convinced that ramping up treatment to the next level is not always the best step to take after a failed cycle or a miscarriage.

las and may trigger mild allergic reactions because it's produced by another person.

Humegon, Pergonal, Repronex **(BioSimilar FSH and LH).** These formulations are extracted and purified from the urine of menopausal women. These are outdated medications, which I rarely prescribe. But they are an option for a limited number of women who don't produce enough LH to adequately trigger the production of estradiol, such as women with anorexia or who have lost pituitary function. *Pros:* They are the cheapest of the injectable medications used to promote egg development. *Cons:* You will need to mix and dilute the medication prior to use. Both Humegon and Pergonal require an intramuscular injection and are therefore difficult to self-administer. They also tend to be less potent than BioIdentical FSH. *My tips: I recommend passing on this outdated and hard-to-use drug and use Menopur, described below, if you don't produce enough LH.*

Menopur **(BioSimilar FSH and LH).** This is a more highly purified form of the BioSimilar preparations above, and also contains a standardized dose of equal amounts of FSH and LH. *Pros:* Since it is highly processed, this treatment is more potent than Humegon, Repronex, and Pergonal. It's also subcutaneous, not intramuscular. *Cons:* You will need to mix and dilute the medication prior to use. It also tends to cost more.

Novarel, Ovidrel, Pregnyl, Profasi (BioSimilar LH). These treatments are typically used to trigger ovulation after one of the FSH products or clomiphene has stimulated your ovaries to produce the desired amount of mature eggs. They are derived from the urine of pregnant women, because their urine contains the hormone HCG, which is a near cookie-cutter copy of LH, the hormone that triggers ovulation. The drug is administered by injection, typically at the doctor's office following your last ultrasound. Most women will ovulate about 36 hours after the injection. Since this hormone circulates in your bloodstream for several days after the injection, it also helps boost early progesterone production by your ovaries following ovulation—an added bonus that assists with implantation. Though using BioSimilar LH is not necessary for ovulation, it's important for the purposes of timing if you're scheduling an insemination or egg retrieval.

Luveris (BioIdentical LH). This product is so new, most fertility specialists are still gaining experience in its use. Although some have already embraced it because it's a BioIdentical hormone and therefore safer than BioSimilar LH, there is some data suggesting that it may not be as effective, but the debate is ongoing. *My tips: Find out why your physician recommends this treatment, as we're still early in the evaluation process of this product.*

Antagon, Cetrotide (BioAntagonist LH). These medications block the release of FSH and LH from your brain to your ovaries. They are typically used to delay ovulation when timing procedures, as well as to reduce the risk of ovarian hyperstimulation syndrome in susceptible women. The treatment involves a daily injection you take beginning around menstrual day 8 or so. *My tips: I have found that by carefully adjusting the dose of the FSH formulations, I have rarely had to use this medication for ovulation induction or enhancement cycles, though I have used them to delay ovulation if a couple learns midcycle that they will be apart during the fertile window and ovulation needs to be delayed. They are used primarily with ART cycles.*

Did you know ?

I have abandoned the use of the term "artificial insemination," the older term for intrauterine insemination, because it implies that we're doing something unnatural rather than trying to enhance natural reproduction.

INTRAUTERINE INSEMINATION

Most fertility specialists recommend intrauterine insemination (IUI) whenever a couple goes through ovulation induction in order to optimize their results at the lowest possible cost. Even if your partner's semen analysis indicates that he is male factor 1, or presumed fertile, it's worth doing insemination to sidestep any unidentified sperm factors, because the semen analysis has limitations and doesn't test how your partner's sperm will interact with your cervix, uterus, or fallopian tubes.

IUI is better than sex because it has a higher success rate. Advances in procedures that prepare the specimen have given it the edge. As I

AN ASSIST FROM VIAGRA

It's not uncommon for a man to have difficulty obtaining an erection, let alone to ejaculate, when he's feeling the pressure of someone waiting for his specimen. Most men are aware of their comfort level and their performance under these circumstances, and fertility clinics accommodate a man's request for a little assistance from erection-enhancing drugs when necessary.

Viagra and the like have become wildly popular over the last 10 years, and most people have become more accustomed to discussing their use for recreation. Unfortunately, fertility clinics don't always think to offer these medications to patients before they schedule an IUI. If your partner is concerned about not being able to provide a specimen, suggest that he discuss this option with your doctor. Of these medications, I recommend Cialis for my patients. It begins to work in as little as 30 minutes and lasts for about 36 hours. As a result, one 10 mg tablet is generally all most men need, even if the plan is for two inseminations.

described in chapter 8, every time a man ejaculates, some of his sperm is very active and healthy, but some of it is dying, and some of it is already dead. And more than half of the sperm are typically abnormal in their appearance. By contrast, when your partner brings his specimen to the fertility center, the process of sperm preparation isolates all of the healthy, active, normal sperm and discards the rest.

Once this elite bunch has been separated, they'll go through a process called *sperm washing.* This involves removing the semen, which contains chemicals that can cause you tremendous cramping if it got inside your uterus (during sex, the semen doesn't get into a woman's uterus, only the sperm do). The sperm will also be bathed in a liquid that enhances their ability to swim toward your awaiting eggs, and protects them from damaging free radicals.

Dr. Greene

Intrauterine insemination has been part of fertility treatment for more than 50 years, but during the early days, there were no good methods for separating the sperm from the semen. So they would place the specimen within a woman's cervix, a process called *intracervical insemination (ICI),* in order to minimize discomfort for the woman and avoid the risk of her developing an infection with the use of IUI. Modern techniques for sperm preparation and the use of special catheters have made IUI a safe, effective, and comfortable procedure. In fact, studies demonstrate that IUI is three to five times more effective than ICI. If you're planning an insemination, my recommendation is for IUI, not ICI.

Finally, the specimen is placed in your uterus using a long, flexible catheter. I am told that this procedure, like a Pap smear, can be a bit uncomfortable but not painful. Within minutes, the sperm will reach the safe haven of the fallopian tubes—with ovulation induction or enhancement, both ovaries ovulate. Some fertility centers will recommend two inseminations performed 24 hours apart, whereas other centers may only suggest one with the plan for you and your partner to have intercourse on the second day. My recommendation varies depending on each couple's unique history. *My tips: I recommend including IUI with any treatment for any female factors that don't require advanced reproductive techniques based on the nomogram (OF1 to OF3, TF1 to TF2 and occasionally TF3, UF1 to UF3, and EF1 to EF2). It's also appropriate for MF1 to*

DONOR INSEMINATION (IUI-D)

If you don't have a male partner or if you and your partner have decided not to use his sperm, you may need to turn to a sperm donor. The sperm bank industry is regulated and monitored by the FDA, so rest assured that every sperm donor is carefully vetted through a process of medical, genetic, and psychological screenings. These banks also limit the number of children produced from any single donor. If you need an anonymous sperm donor, ask your health care provider to recommend a company. I encourage my patients to contact California Cryobank (www.cryobank.com). They have been around for over 30 years and are truly a full-service organization with an impeccable reputation. Sperm can be shipped cross-country.

MF2, as well as MF3, if at least 5 million actively swimming sperm can be isolated from your specimen through sperm washing. If not, you're better off considering ART options as your first line of treatment.

LUTEAL SUPPORT

There is very little data on the necessity of *luteal support,* the supplementation of progesterone to help make the endometrium fertile, following ovulation induction or enhancement. Therefore, most fertility specialists make recommendations based upon their personal opinion and their own interpretation of the available science. One thing we know is that the pattern of hormone fluctuations of even the most fertile women can vary substantially from month to month, so anyone can experience luteal phase deficiency at one time or another. When you add the hormone-tipping effects of the different medications used during OI treatment, it stands to reason that many women may need a boost of progesterone to balance out the effects of unnaturally high estradiol levels on the endometrium. The goal is to minimize hormone imbalances in order to reduce the chance of multiple pregnancies. Progesterone and estradiol work in a yin and yang fashion. Lower progesterone levels (less than 20 ng/ml) during the week following ovulation are associated with a significantly lower rate of successful implantation.

I individualize my recommendation for each patient based upon her history, her treatment, and her preference. Since the science can't provide definitive guidelines, discuss luteal support thoroughly with your doctor. If you do decide to use some supplementation, I would encourage you to use an FDA-approved BioIdentical preparation to avoid any possible adverse effect upon your child. BioIdentical progesterone is indistinguishable from the progesterone made by your body and won't cause any problems aside from the common side effects of progesterone—bloating, breast tenderness, constipation, and fatigue.

> *Prometrium* (BioIdentical progesterone) is a capsule that is available in 100 mg or 200 mg doses. Your dose can be adjusted to keep your level above 20 ng/ml for at least two weeks after insemination, at which time a pregnancy test can be performed to confirm whether you're pregnant. *My tips: I prefer this form of progesterone for women that need luteal support. If you're allergic to peanuts, however, this is not for you since it is contained in a peanut oil base. If you feel overly fatigued, dizzy, or have unacceptable mood changes on this medication, I recommend that you try using the capsule vaginally. It will be absorbed in your uterus but less will get to your brain to trigger symptoms.*

> *Crinone, Prochieve, and Endometrin* (BioIdentical progesterone) are vaginal preparations inserted with an applicator. For women who experience excessive symptoms from progesterone tablets, this method tends to be more easily tolerated. *My tips: The disadvantage is that blood tests are not accurate in assessing whether your dose is sufficient. Research shows that with a gel, much more progesterone is absorbed into the uterine lining than is measurable in the bloodstream. This product also tends to cost more than the capsules.*

KNOWING WHEN IT'S TIME TO MOVE ON

You haven't wasted time if you've learned something from a treatment that wasn't successful. I recommend you start out with the least expensive treatment that is appropriate for your situation—based on your fertility factors and the nomogram on page 225. Once you choose your course of action, try to commit to at least three legitimate attempts before you move on; the data shows that on your third attempt, your statistical chance of success is as high as it was on your first attempt. But with your fourth, fifth, and sixth attempts, your success rate becomes lower and lower. For instance, once you have ovulated on clomiphene, complete three cycles, and then consider whether you'd like to try one or two more cycles or move on to advanced reproductive treatments. If, however, you fail to ovulate on clomiphene alone, at least you've learned that you are clomiphene resistant and you can consider a combination therapy or move on to the more potent injectable medications.

Periodically, it's worthwhile to sit down with your fertility specialist and review your plan if it hasn't succeeded. Consider whether some fertility factor may not have been thoroughly evaluated. If so, it may be time to move on to the advanced reproductive techniques in the next chapter.

14 Advanced Reproductive Treatments

In the last 30 years, 3 million children have been born in the United States with the help of ART. Because of their success and growing popularity, these procedures are no longer thought of as the last-ditch effort for desperate couples, but part of the process of having children when the earlier steps weren't successful. But sometimes their highly publicized success rates also attract couples to the advanced procedures before they have exhausted their less-invasive options. Too many people choose ART based upon feelings of desperation mixed with the urgency to get pregnant, rather than need. I want to remind you that the majority of couples can achieve pregnancy through hormone balance and basic fertility treatments. Having said that, I do recognize that some couples do need ART to become pregnant. My goal in this chapter is to improve your understanding of these high-tech procedures, as well as focus on the benefits of hormone balance as a complement to ART—to lower your expense, improve your pregnancy rate, and maximize your chance of having a healthy baby.

IVF: THE BIRTH OF A NEW TECHNOLOGY

Since 1978, when the first "test tube baby" was conceived in a petri dish in England, treating infertility has grown into an entire industry. In 2006, there were more than 400 IVF clinics in the United States that performed nearly 110,000 procedures. It's estimated that about 1 of every 80 American babies is born as a result of IVF today.

Since the inception of IVF, success rates have grown steadily. In 1996, when fertility centers were first required to start reporting their success rates to a central agency, the live birth rate was 28 percent, and in 2004, it had risen to 34 percent. The statistics show, however, that by 2002, success rates reached a plateau, but there has been continued improvement in certain subgroups of patients as procedures have become more refined. For example, in women younger than 35, the live birth rate was highest at 53 percent per embryo transfer when only two embryos were transferred per cycle, suggesting that efforts to lower the multiple birth rate by using fewer embryos may also improve success rates. We're finding that success rates may improve further as we get better at nurturing embryos in the laboratory and develop techniques that allow us to select the healthiest one or two for transfer.

> ## Did you know
>
> Less than 15 percent of couples with infertility need ART to achieve their goal of having their own biologic children.

ART: THE TREATMENTS

There are many different types of ART, as evidenced by the alphabet soup of acronyms, below. Your options may be limited to those prac-

BEING ACCOUNTABLE

Today, ART are under the regulatory supervision of the CDC with the assistance of the Society for Assisted Reproductive Technology (SART). The rapid growth and competition between fertility centers led Congress to pass the Fertility Clinic Success Rate and Certification Act of 1992, resulting in independent oversight of quality control and monitoring advertised success rates. Today, every cycle is reported at its initiation and followed to completion by this joint organization to ensure the accuracy of reported live birth rates resulting from today's technology. The most current results, from 2004, including the specific results of each clinic, are available at http://www.cdc.gov/art.

ticed by your fertility center, but try to familiarize yourself with each procedure so you have a broad idea of what is available.

IVF (in vitro fertilization). Though refined over the years, IVF remains essentially the same as it did 30 years ago. You go through a preparatory cycle in which your ovaries are first suppressed in order to gain control of the hormones, followed by ovulation enhancement to get as many healthy eggs to mature as possible. When your response has peaked, you are given an injection to simulate the LH signal for the eggs to complete their final step of maturation—to divide their chromosomes from 46 to 23, so that they can combine with your partner's sperm. Then, prior to ovulation, a procedure is scheduled to retrieve each egg from your ovaries using a long needle under the guidance of an ultrasound. These eggs are then placed in a petri dish along with a defined number of prepared sperm (typically 25,000 to 50,000) from your partner. They are suspended in a nutrient solution that simulates the fluid inside a healthy fallopian tube and left to incubate in a reduced oxygen environment. After 16 to 20 hours, they are removed and examined for signs of fertilization. A fertilized egg (zygote) has two distinct yolklike structures called *pronuclei.* Each zygote is then placed back into the incubator until it is transferred into the woman's uterus via a procedure called embryo transfer (see page 250) or frozen and stored for a future pregnancy. *My tips: IVF is a necessity for women with TF4 since it is the only way for sperm and egg to meet. I also recommend it for women with EF3 or EF4, but if you've failed to conceive after 4 to 6 attempts of ovulation induction or enhancement with IUI, then this is your next step regardless of your factors, even if you only have MF1, OF1, TF1, and UF1.*

GIFT (gamete intrafallopian transfer) This procedure skips the petri dish and simply takes the eggs retrieved from a woman's ovary and transfers them along with her partner's sperm directly into her fallopian tubes. It gained popularity in the late 1980s when incubation techniques weren't as effective, and made up about 25 percent of ART procedures at the time. The success rates actually exceeded those of IVF until about 1995, when IVF started becoming more successful. I don't recommend GIFT; today, it's more expensive and more invasive than IVF, because it requires a laparoscopy to place eggs and sperm into the fallopian tubes. Although the success rates remain steady at 35 to 40 percent (in women 35 or younger), less than 1 percent of today's ART procedures involve GIFT. In 2005, only 340 GIFT procedures were performed in the United States.

ET (embryo transfer). This is the final step in an IVF treatment. By the second or third day after fertilization, each embryo consists of 4 to 10 cells clustered together in a solid bunch, like a microscopic raspberry. It still contains the zona pellucida, the tough membrane. Depending on your age and the appearance of the embryos, your physician will place one to three of the embryos into a soft sterile catheter and transfer them into your womb. This painless procedure is similar to a Pap smear in that a speculum is placed in the vagina to expose your cervix. The soft catheter is then gently passed up into the womb, and with a tiny amount of fluid, the embryos are transferred into the endometrium. *My tips: Many centers perform ET under guidance from an ultrasound to place the embryo in the best possible position in your uterus. Accumulating evidence suggests that this does improve implantation rates.*

Ask Dr. Greene

Q Can I get pain medication during my egg retrieval?

A Most IVF centers provide pain medication to patients that request it and, quite frankly, most patients do. Although the procedure typically takes only 10 to 15 minutes, it can be painful, and it's important that you remain still. For these reasons, I typically recommend a short-acting general anesthesia, but some centers only offer either a local anesthesia or intravenous pain medication or both.

ICSI (intracytoplasmic sperm injection). Several adaptations of basic IVF have been developed, broadening the list of problems that can be treated by ART. ICSI (pronounced ick-see) was the first successful procedure created to treat severe male factor infertility (male factor 4). In standard IVF, thousands of sperm are placed near the egg in a petri dish and the penetration of the egg is allowed to occur without assistance. In ICSI, a single healthy sperm is physically placed under the hard shell, or zona pellucida, of each egg to promote fertilization. ICSI was originally developed for men with problems such as a previous vasectomy, absence of the vas deferens,

our story

Robert: When we were planning our ART cycle, our fertility specialist, buoyed by his center's success with ICSI, enthusiastically encouraged us to add ICSI to our planned cycle. We didn't have any diagnosed male factor issues, and weren't true candidates for the procedure. As a colleague, I said no thanks. I explained that it would provide useful diagnostic information to see if Morgan's eggs would fertilize without ICSI, and might provide guidance for future cycles. He respected our decision, and we moved forward with standard IVF.

exceptionally low sperm count, and poor morphology or motility, or for couples that had a previous IVF cycle without any of the eggs being successfully fertilized. Fertility centers have become so skillful at selecting sperm and performing this procedure without damaging the egg that today about 80 percent of eggs injected develop into embryos. But because of its success, some centers use it in 50 to 80 percent of all cycles, even in the absence of a male factor. Be aware that not all couples need it, and it's not likely to improve your success rate if you don't need it.

ICSI comes with a few risks. About 5 percent of the eggs retrieved become damaged during sperm insertion and will not develop. There's also a slightly increased risk of having a child with an abnormality of the sex chromosomes, X or Y. This occurs in 0.8 percent (8 per 1,000) of children born through ICSI, compared to 0.2 percent (2 per 1,000) of children born through standard IVF. Although the exact reason for this increased risk is uncertain, it is widely believed that it is caused by a subtle genetic abnormality in the sperm, as men with male factor 4, who are offered this procedure, have a higher incidence of these abnormalities. It is also possible that the procedure itself may contribute to this disorder.

I recommend preconception counseling for all couples undergoing ICSI. Men with congenital bilateral absence of the vas deferens (CBAVD), in particular, should get genetic testing for cystic fibrosis. If you and your partner carry one of several genetic abnormalities that cause cystic fibrosis, you are more likely to have a child with this disorder if you're using ICSI. *My tips: The enthusiasm over*

Case in Point

Isabelle, 34, had suffered for nearly 10 years with endometriosis and endured endless cycles of pain, surgery, and other attempts to control the disease. By the time I first met her and her husband, Simon, 37, she had undergone five surgeries and three courses of Lupron, the ovarian suppression drug that causes symptoms of menopause, but her pain had returned. They came to my office because they wanted to become pregnant, and she was considering a hysterectomy following her delivery to resolve her discomfort.

After reviewing their records and tests, I saw that Isabelle's ovarian reserve was diminished by her multiple surgeries. Her endometriosis had been stage 3 (moderate) at the time of her last surgery. They had never used contraception during their 10 years together, but had never conceived. They also had acknowledged that their sex life was frequently interrupted when Isabelle's endometriosis was at its worst. I performed an ultrasound, which confirmed that Isabelle's fallopian tubes were swollen and filled with fluid. She also had what appeared to be an *endometrioma*—a cluster of endometriosis within her ovary. I suggested that they should consider having me perform yet another laparoscopy, but this time I would not only remove the endometriosis, including the endometrioma in her ovaries to improve the quality of her eggs, but I would remove her fallopian tubes. Based upon her history, she would need IVF to become pregnant, so removing her diseased tubes would improve the ability of embryos to implant. After much thought, they decided to proceed. Her surgery went well, but it took me nearly five hours to work through her extensive (stage 4) endometriosis and the scar tissue caused by the disorder and the prior surgeries.

I placed her on a birth control pill for three months to give her ovaries a period of rest. After her recovery, she felt remarkably well. She began a prenatal vitamin, a DHA supplement, and started the Perfect Balance program. She took additional steps to reduce her exposure to BioMutagens from plastics and cosmetics, to lower her chance of a recurrence. At that point, she and Simon were eager to proceed with the IVF cycle.

Her ovulation enhancement went well and we retrieved eight eggs. We had planned to do ICSI on half of them, since they were concerned about them not fertilizing. Two of them did fertilize without ICSI and three did with ICSI. They transferred two embryos and had the other three cryopreserved. They delivered twins three years ago. Their embryos are still in cold storage, and Isabelle felt well enough that she chose not to undergo a hysterectomy.

ICSI has resulted in its overuse. The couples who can truly benefit are those with MF4 or couples that have previously experienced fertilization failure (see page 265 for more information on the overuse of ICSI).

ICSI spin-offs. As ICSI has evolved, several techniques have been developed for obtaining sperm in men who aren't able to ejaculate even a few hundred sperm. These are the male equivalents of an egg retrieval, and are often used instead of reversing a vasectomy or in men whose vas deferens are blocked or absent since birth. These procedures can be performed ahead of time, freezing sperm until the egg retrieval has been performed or for future pregnancies. Some urologists, when performing a vasectomy reversal, will also do one of these techniques as insurance in case normal sperm aren't ejaculated after the surgery. Here is a brief description of the procedures available. They are generally performed by a urologist specially trained in reproductive endocrinology.

- *MESA (microsurgical epididymal sperm aspiration).* A small needle is placed through a mini incision guided by a microscope to withdraw (aspirate) sperm from the epididymis, the holding room of sperm. It is performed in an operating room under local or general anesthesia by a urologist with microsurgery skills. Sperm are very concentrated in this location, so even a trace amount of fluid will typically yield more than a million sperm. MESA is associated with the highest pregnancy rates and has the lowest risk, but it tends to be significantly more expensive and therefore should only be used when necessary.

- *PESA (percutaneous epididymal sperm aspiration)* is also fast and can be done simply with a local anesthetic, rather than general anesthesia. It does not require an incision because the surgeon simply inserts the aspirating needle into the epididymis, finding it by palpating the skin rather than using a microscope. Typically, fewer sperm are retrieved than with MESA, and there is a slight risk of developing a harmless but potentially uncomfortable *hematoma,* a collection of blood at the injection site—the equivalent of a "black-and-blue" mark of the scrotum.

- *TESE (testicular sperm extraction).* This procedure is an alternative to MESA and PESA—and may be the only option your local provider offers. During a surgical procedure in the operating room under local anesthesia with IV sedation, a small incision is made to expose the testis, and sperm are obtained through several small biopsies. TESE may also be diagnostic if it is uncertain why the male partner is not producing sperm. This procedure does not obtain as many sperm as the ones that target the epididymis.

- *TESA (testicular sperm aspiration)* is an adaptation of TESE that simply uses a needle placed through the scrotum into the testicle without making an incision first. This procedure is quick and can typically be accomplished with a local anesthetic. Although it can be easily repeated, it does yield fewer sperm and can result in hematoma.

AH (assisted hatching). This procedure is sometimes offered to couples who have had two or more failed IVF attempts or for women older than 38. It is believed that one reason more women don't get pregnant after an IVF cycle is because of a failure of the embryo to hatch out of the zona pellucida. Normally, an embryo breaks free from this protective shell in about 120 hours after fertilization, a step that allows it to implant in the endometrium. AH involves creating an opening in the zona pellucida to make it easier for the embryo to emerge. AH is typically performed on day 3 after fertilization. It comes with the risk of creating a lethal injury to the embryo as well as a slight increased risk of having identical (monozygotic) twins— about two to three times higher than the normal rate of 0.3 percent, or 3 sets per every 1,000 deliveries. AH can produce twins if a single cell or a small group of cells gets through the opening and begins multiplying, setting up the potential to develop two genetically identical embryos. *My tips: This procedure is an important add-on for women over 38, who tend to have a tougher zona pellucida. There is some evidence that younger women with diminished ovarian reserve can also benefit from this procedure. If you're considering AH, ask about the experience, success rates, and technique used by your fertility center, as results vary considerably. Several techniques are available.*

- *Mechanical AH* was the first technique developed in 1990. Under a powerful microscope, a tiny glass needle is used to create a narrow slit in the zona pellucida.

- *Chemical thinning.* A very weak acid solution, called Tyrode, is used to thin the zona pellucida. The acid is applied to an area as far away from the developing embryo as possible to avoid injury, and then is promptly washed away. This procedure is performed under a powerful microscope and creates a larger hole than the mechanical method, which may reduce the risk of identical twinning.
- *Laser-assisted hatching.* This latest evolution has been shown to result in the highest pregnancy rate of these methods. It is also the easiest to perform, with the lowest risk of injury to the embryo since there is no contact. As it does involve extra equipment, however, it is more costly.

PGD (preimplantation genetic diagnosis). This most recent development in ART allows couples to test their embryos for chromosomal abnormalities prior to transferring them into the woman's uterus. This test involves removing one of the 6 to 10 cells present in each embryo on day 3 after fertilization. The removed cell can be tested for an extra or missing chromosome. Currently, tests exist for 9 of the 24 chromosomes (13, 15, 16, 17, 18, 21, 22, X, and Y), which allows screening for the most commonly inherited chromosome abnormalities, including Down syndrome and Turner's syndrome. There is also a growing number of genetic tests for specific disorders that don't involve a complete loss of or gain of a chromosome, such as cystic fibrosis, Tay-Sachs disease, sickle-cell anemia, Huntington's disease, fragile X syndrome, myotonic dystrophy, and thalassemia. PGD can significantly reduce the risk of early pregnancy loss in couples with recurrent miscarriage by identifying genetically abnormal embryos and discarding them, rather than transferring them. While PGD is growing in popularity, currently less than 10 percent of centers offer the procedure, and it can add several thousand dollars to the cost of fertility treatment. *My tips: My concern is that as PGD becomes more widely available, it may become a standard part of treatment rather than an option to those who truly need genetic testing.*

Cryopreservation allows couples to store tissue in order to extend their reproductive years, coordinate procedures, or lengthen the life of embryos. In 1949, sperm was the first tissue that was frozen and

SEX SELECTION

PGD has made it possible to select the sex of your new baby, an advance that has raised ethical concerns for some people. There are several reasons why couples might choose the gender. Certainly, some cultures or families put a greater value on one gender over the other. But, more commonly, this request arises when a couple already has a child or children of one sex and would like to select the other for the purposes of "family balancing." Another reason is medical; certain inherited conditions only affect one sex, like Duchenne muscular dystrophy or hemophilia, so if a couple has an inherited condition, choosing the other sex will minimize, if not remove, the risk of the disorder. The ethics boards of ASRM and ACOG support the use of sex selection for the purpose of preventing serious genetic disorders that are linked to a person's sex.

PGD is one method of sex selection. Another still investigational one is called *sperm sorting*. Since the X chromosome is larger and heavier than the Y chromosome, it is possible to select the heavier "female potential" sperm for use in combination with ICSI. There have been several reports of success using this technology, but it is not guaranteed.

thawed to successfully create a pregnancy. Today, sperm cryopreservation is available at most fertility centers. Sperm are technically easy to freeze because they have very little water inside; water expands as it freezes, and in so doing destroys cells, unless they have been dehydrated prior to or during the freezing process.

Embryo and egg freezing. Thirty-five years later, in 1984, the first embryo was frozen and successfully thawed. Today, embryo freezing is available at most fertility centers as a routine part of IVF. Any healthy embryos that are not transferred into a woman's uterus can be frozen and stored in liquid nitrogen at 196°C. Embryos need a cryoprotectant, a media that is used to dehydrate them in the freezing process. Typically, 50 to 75 percent of embryos survive the process of freezing and thawing. To date, embryos have been frozen for up to 13 years before being thawed and transferred to create a pregnancy without any apparent increase in birth defects.

Oocyte freezing involves harvesting and freezing eggs for later maturation and fertilization. This is one option for women who have been diagnosed with cancer or those who want to delay childbearing so they can have their frozen eggs as a backup in case they face fertility challenges when they're ready to have children. Because eggs contain so much water, they are much harder to freeze without causing damage. Even with the use of a cryoprotectant, many of the eggs do not survive the process of freezing and thawing. Yet new techniques are becoming more successful. At the time of this publication, an estimated 150 pregnancies have resulted in healthy babies through this technology. *My tips: Although oocyte freezing tends to be less expensive and it has the added benefit of not requiring the patients to choose a sperm donor, the uncertainty of the current techniques is a drawback. I recommend embryo freezing. But a newer rapid freezing method, called oocyte vitrification, reduces the chance of ice crystals forming and may help overcome prior limitations. Talk to your health care provider about this emerging option.*

Case in Point

Lucy, a successful oncology surgeon, began to think about her own ovarian reserve after counseling a cancer patient about her options to preserve her fertility. As a single woman in a competitive field, she didn't want to slow her career advancement, but, at 35, she remained acutely aware of her dwindling supply of fertile eggs. Concerned with the possibility that she might not marry any time in the near future, and knowing that she couldn't make the sacrifices of being a single mother right now, Lucy decided to consider a more high-tech route. We discussed her options, which were either freezing her eggs or having her eggs fertilized by donor sperm and freezing the resulting embryos. Freezing eggs has a lower success rate, so she decided to do IVF and use an anonymous sperm donor, which resulted in 11 healthy embryos. We froze all of the embryos, giving her some fertility insurance as she pursues her career for several more years, before starting a family.

FET (frozen embryo transfer). When a woman is ready to have a frozen embryo transferred and thawed, she uses FET. She is first placed on a programmed cycle of estradiol and then progesterone in order to prepare her uterus for implantation. When an ultrasound establishes that her endometrium is ready, a prearranged number of embryos are thawed. Most couples choose two or three embryos (if they have that many). If the first thawed embryos don't

NEW HOPE FOR WOMEN WITH CANCER

In 2006, nearly 55,000 women younger than 40 were diagnosed with cancer. Survival rates for the most common cancers, like breast cancer, are very high, and many women can go on to have children. But many chemotherapy agents can cause DNA mutations and premature ovarian failure, major obstacles to fertility.

In the past, there was the concern that a pregnancy could promote the recurrence of breast cancer in survivors, but the latest studies conclude that for most survivors, pregnancy does not worsen their prognosis. Still, women are told to wait at least two years after completing treatment for breast cancer before becoming pregnant. A 2007 study, however, called this conservative recommendation into question. The study revealed that if women with localized disease (not metastasized) became pregnant only six months after completing treatment, it did not adversely affect their prognosis. Based on this research, pregnancy no longer appears to be harmful for women with localized breast cancer that has been treated. But the treatment itself may become their greatest obstacle to conception.

If you've been diagnosed with breast cancer, there is often a two- to three-month gap between surgery and chemotherapy. If you have time, talk to your doctor about whether you're a candidate to go through an IVF cycle to create frozen embryos prior to chemotherapy. These can be stored as fertility insurance in case you experience premature ovarian failure. If you don't have the time, you might want to consider oocyte freezing. In addition, there's one other procedure that is still experimental but has been successful in a handful of pregnancies. It's called *ovarian tissue freezing*. This technique involves using a laparoscopy to remove a section of an ovary. The section is then cut into smaller strips and frozen. When you are ready, the sections can be transplanted back into your body. Currently, the technique still requires ART to stimulate the ovaries and fertilization in the laboratory. Researchers are also investigating the removal, storage, and subsequent replacement of the entire ovary, but this is a more challenging procedure. Although these procedures are still considered experimental, technology moves quickly in the field of reproductive medicine, so ask about the status of these options.

survive, some couples choose to continue thawing embryos and have each embryo checked for viability as it's thawed, until their desired number has been reached.

In 2004, there were 18,560 FET cycles performed in the United States, representing 14 percent of all ART procedures. Nationally, the live birth rate for FET was nearly 28 percent. Although that was about 6 percent lower than the pregnancy rate for fresh embryo transfers, the cost of an FET is about one-third the cost of an IVF procedure because the steps of egg stimulation, egg retrieval, and fertilization were completed during the original IVF procedure that produced the extra embryos. Ask your fertility center about their success rate for FET, since rates vary considerably. I have had several patients that were fortunate enough to have two or more successful pregnancies from one IVF cycle. After IVF, they implanted several fresh embryos, resulting in a successful pregnancy; later on, they thawed the frozen embryos to have one or more successful pregnancies using FET.

WEIGHING THE RISKS OF ART

Most couples are attracted to ART because it's generally faster at achieving pregnancy compared to other options. But it comes with a price tag. The average cost of ART is nearly $14,000 per cycle—cost varies according to how much medication is needed and which add-on procedures, such as ICSI, embryo freezing, or genetic testing, are performed. There are other costs that may be even more important to consider—such as the potential complications of ART.

Ovarian hyperstimulation syndrome. OHSS is the most serious and common complication of ART, a result of the high doses of FSH that are used to coax numerous eggs to maturation. Occurring in up to 5 percent of cycles, OHSS causes ovarian swelling, pelvic pain, increased risk of blood clots, and the accumulation of fluid in the abdomen. It may require hospitalization (see page 237 for more information on risk factors and symptoms). Although OHSS usually indicates that a pregnancy has been achieved (great news!), it must be managed carefully in order to prevent serious health risks.

Multiple gestations. Having a multiple pregnancy is one of the most common complications of ART, and yet it may be the most preventable. Of the ART pregnancies that occurred in 2004, 30 percent were twins and 3 percent were triplets. These numbers are still too high. In the beginning, the low success rates of IVF motivated fertility experts to transfer more embryos. But as the techniques for culturing embryos

Dr. Greene

Certain women at high risk of OHSS can reduce their risk by as much as 70 percent if they receive an injection of a protein called albumin. A 25 to 50 gram dose is injected at the time of their egg retrieval. You may be considered high risk if you have PCOS, you're using high doses of FSH, you're less than 25 years old, you're below normal weight, or you've had OHSS in the past. Talk to your doctor about whether you should be given this treatment to reduce your risk of OHSS. After your egg retrieval, stay well hydrated by drinking at least one liter of an electrolyte supplemented drink per day. See page 237 for warning signs of OHSS.

improved, so did success rates, making these older motivations no longer applicable. We're now seeing the beginning of a trend to lower the number of embryos transferred. Still, fertility centers have had difficulty educating their patients of the potential benefits of reducing the number of embryos transferred, despite the recent research showing that it may not reduce their success rate, and may even improve it. In 2006, the ASRM teamed up with ACOG and the March of Dimes to urge women going through fertility treatment to take steps to reduce the incidence of preterm births caused by multiple gestations.

Preterm labor and other pregnancy complications. Attempting to reduce your chance of a multiple pregnancy will significantly lower your risk of preterm birth. But if you've conceived through ART, even if you are carrying only one baby, you still have twice the risk of preterm delivery or of having a baby that is small for its gestational age. You're also at high risk of gestational diabetes and preeclampsia, a potentially life-threatening disorder of pregnancy. Although the relationship between ART and these complications has not been clearly established, I believe that the hormonal manipulations of treatment contribute to these problems; each of these pregnancy complications has been linked to specific hormonal imbalances. But by carefully monitoring your pregnancy and paying attention to your symptoms, you can lower your risks of these problems. Once you're pregnant, talk to your OB about all the ways your diet and lifestyle can improve the outcome of your pregnancy and the health of your baby. I'd also recommend you refer to my book *Perfect Hormone Balance for Pregnancy* to help balance your hormones and lower these elevated risks.

Birth defects. There is a slight increase in the rate of birth defects in IVF babies compared to those conceived through other fertility treatments and those conceived without any treatment. The largest study suggested that 6.2 percent of IVF children in the United States had a congenital malformation, compared to 4.5 percent of those conceived without this treatment. Whether this effect is real or the result of closer scrutiny of babies born through IVF is uncertain. It has also been suggested that some couples who require ART may have mild genetic abnormalities that have contributed to their infertility—these gene defects may be responsible for the increased incidence of birth defects in this group.

IMPROVING YOUR ART SUCCESS

ART success rates reached a plateau several years ago. At the same time, there is still an inordinately high risk of twins, putting women and their babies at risk of complications. But at the forefront of the fertility world, experts are using techniques that both push success rates higher and lower complication rates. For these techniques to be the most effective, you need to correct hormonal imbalances prior to initiating ART, as well as try to reduce the way ovarian stimulation hormones disrupt your hormone balance. The Perfect Balance Fertility Program addresses how you can achieve hormone balance. Here, I'll describe the techniques and approaches that can improve your success rates even more.

Transfer one embryo. Fueled by the goal of reducing the incidence of risky multiple births, many countries have passed laws limiting the number of embryos permitted for transfer to one per treatment cycle, called *single embryo transfer (SET)*. By comparison, in the United States, SET was used in only 8 percent of ART cycles, and four or more embryos were transferred in 21 percent of ART cycles. In other countries, these government mandates have created a strong motivation among fertility specialists to investigate ways to maximize pregnancy rates with only one embryo. They've improved techniques in the laboratory, such as the type of media used to culture embryos. We can benefit by applying what they've learned and by voluntarily taking the same precautionary steps.

EXPERIMENTAL IMMUNOLOGICAL TREATMENT

Over the last several years, some fertility clinics have claimed that antiphospholipid antibodies may be hindering implantation during ART (I explain their use in the section on recurrent miscarriage; see page 214). In 1999, the ASRM Practice Committee recommended *against* the use of these immunological treatments in ART, based on a comprehensive review. In 2006, they reviewed more current data and confirmed their earlier guidelines. If your provider recommends treating antiphospholipid antibodies, ask him if any new evidence supports his advice or check with www.asrm.org to see if they have modified their guidelines.

One report on women between the ages of 36 and 39 who electively chose to do SET demonstrated a pregnancy rate of 54 percent and a live birth rate of 42 percent, but those who had two embryos transferred had a pregnancy rate of 35 percent with a live birth rate of 27 percent. I encourage you to consider, if all prognostic signs look good, having only one embryo transferred and freezing the rest for FET if you do not become pregnant.

Individualize ovarian stimulation. Several studies suggest that using lower doses of ovarian stimulation medication yields fewer, albeit higher-quality, eggs. This approach dovetails nicely with the movement toward transferring only one or two embryos. Mild to moderate stimulation may deliver higher-quality oocytes because it recruits the ones most likely to fertilize and result in a pregnancy. Indeed, milder stimulation more closely mimics the body's physiology than aggressive high-dose stimulation and forced egg maturation. These lower doses also reduce your risk of complications, such as OHSS and thyroid disturbances that can increase the risk of miscarriage. The dose you'll need can be predicted in part by your fertility factors and in part by your previous response to medications. Discuss with your physician ways to individualize your dose of medications to yield the highest-quality eggs and improve your chance of successful treatment.

Blastocyst transfer. In a naturally conceived pregnancy, an embryo does not arrive into the uterus until it has grown to 16 to 32 cells, the *blastocyst* stage, after having spent about five days multiplying in the fallopian tube. But with IVF, it's difficult to keep embryos alive in the laboratory past day 3, so multiple embryos were transferred early and we hoped for the best. Over the last several years, however, culture techniques have improved, allowing embryos to be cultured until the blastocyst stage—day 5. While some centers offer blastocyst transfer, many centers are reluctant to do it since it increases the risk that none of the embryos will survive to day 5 for transfer, a disappointing moment for couples. Yet evidence suggests that these blastocysts may not have survived in the womb either, as up to 40 percent of day 3 embryos may have a chromosomal anomaly that will become apparent and result in demise by day 5. In other words, centers may be transferring potentially damaged embryos before the damage is visible. Yet in women less than 35 years of age, implantation rates and live birth rates are twice as high when a blastocyst is transferred compared to an embryo. The 2004 SART report demonstrated that a day 5 blastocyst had a higher live birth rate for every age category. In that year, blastocysts were transferred in only 21 percent of the cycles performed in the United States. Consider asking your fertility specialist if you're a candidate for blastocyst transfer, and if you do it, only transfer one (two at the most) to keep your multiple pregnancy risk as low as possible.

Comparative genomic hybridization (CGH). This is a novel technique that is only being performed by some labs. CGH provides a way to assess the entire genetic code of an embryo to ensure that it's normal before selecting it for embryo transfer. This technique has the potential to double current success rates. Currently, embryos are selected based upon their appearance under the microscope, which doesn't reveal anything about their chromosomes. When preimplantation genetic diagnosis (PGD) is added to the process using the most common technique, called FISH, it can identify some specific abnormalities, but it can only test up to 12 chromosomes, and it has not been shown to increase the success rate of IVF. A 2007 study demonstrated that two-thirds of human eggs have subtle genetic damage that limits their ability to form a normal embryo. By selecting a normal embryo through CGH, you can reduce the risk of miscarriage, multiple births, and chromosomal birth defects while increasing the

CONSIDER WEIGHT LOSS BEFORE ART

If you're overweight or obese, and younger than 35, consider losing weight before attempting ART treatment. Several studies have demonstrated that the hormonal imbalance associated with excess abdominal weight may be your greatest obstacle to success—even with high-tech treatment. Women younger than 30 with a BMI of 35 or higher may be diminishing their chance of a live birth by up to 50 percent. Talk to your doctor about whether you'd be a good candidate for insulin-sensitizing therapy like metformin. Follow my nutrition and exercise plan, and work with a nutritionist to lose at least 5 percent of your total body weight over the next three months. Not only will your chance of success improve, but you stand to save a considerable amount of money by avoiding repeat cycles of ART.

chance for implantation. CGH even reduces the need for genetic testing during pregnancy.

Reduce stress. In the first 25 years of ART, more than 700 articles and studies were published on the complex and multilayered relationship between emotions and IVF. The sheer interest in this demonstrates how big a role stress plays in fertility. The fertility challenge itself is a source of stress—going through treatment can be all-consuming and stressful, the cost can add financial stress, and the uncertainty of the outcome adds a huge element of anxiety to the mix. Add to the stress cocktail the high estrogen levels that result from fertility treatments and you can make the brain more susceptible to anxiety, which can trigger a cascade of hormonal shifts that may lead to chronic stress and reduce your chance of becoming pregnant.

Review the stress-reducing methods described in the Perfect Balance program. This is a good time to practice meditation and relaxation exercises. Keep in mind that stress levels tend to spike around key events related to treatment cycles, such as around the time of egg retrieval or embryo transfer. Studies demonstrate that acupuncture may reduce stress hormone levels and improve treatment outcome—especially when performed during these critical times. If you're interested in acupuncture, ask your fertility specialist for a referral.

Think twice about ICSI. In 2004, nearly 60 percent of cycles included this fertilization-enhancing procedure, even though half of the couples did not have a male factor high enough to justify it. I believe that many of these procedures were included simply out of fear of fertilization failure. Since ICSI is unlikely to improve your success rate if you don't need it, and it may cause a small increase in the risk of congenital problems, don't feel pressured to accept this add-on procedure. On the other hand, it may be beneficial to consider ICSI as a way of overcoming problems related to a hormone imbalance, such as low sperm count or poor egg quality. For men with male factor 3 or women with reduced ovarian reserve, ICSI can improve the chance of fertilization in ways that restoring hormone balance may not be able to accomplish. If you do have ICSI, you can reduce the chance of having a damaged embryo transferred if you have preimplantation genetic diagnosis. If you're uncertain about what to do, request a "split" procedure. This would involve performing ICSI on half of the oocytes and having the others fertilized through the traditional technique. If you don't conceive through standard IVF and decide to do another cycle, you'll have more information about your fertilization rates to help you decide if you want to try ICSI the second time around. If your oocytes fertilized fine without ICSI, save the money and lower your risk the next time around.

Aggressive luteal support is a means of monitoring your endometrium to see if it's ready for implantation and adjusting your hormone treatment accordingly. ART cycles, in which the ovary is suppressed, and then stimulated, are so different from naturally occurring ones that they require careful supervision and monitoring. Most fertility centers are aggressive about how they manage your ovarian stimulation, yet become very passive once they have embryos in the laboratory. By using an ultrasound to measure the thickness of your endometrial lining while you're on ovarian stimulation medications, your doctor can assess whether your uterus is on schedule for implantation. According to one study, if the endometrium was at least 16 mm thick, the live birth rate was 68 percent, but it dropped to 45 percent if it was only 8 mm thick. Ask your fertility specialist to measure your endometrial thickness during every ultrasound after day 10 of your cycle. If your endometrium is less than 8 mm, discuss whether you may have a

Case in Point

Gita and Mark were at the peak of their economic success and enjoying their second marriage each. Gita was 51 and had four grown children. Mark was 45 and had never fathered a child. They had been together for about five years before they came to my office to discuss having a child together.

Because of Gita's age, I explained that their best option was to use an egg donor. Gita was very healthy, and Mark was also very fit and active, and took a medication to reduce his cholesterol. They proposed using Gita's 35-year-old niece as the egg donor. I understood their desire to keep the egg in the family, but I cautioned against using a family member (or a friend), as I had seen too many similar situations deteriorate. We typically recommend semianonymous egg donors—women in their early to mid 20s who have indicated their desire to undergo ovulation enhancement and egg retrieval with minimal contact with the recipient couple. We coordinate their care through an agency experienced in performing all the genetic and psychological screening of donors, as well as handling the legal considerations.

After some thought, they agreed. They decided to work with an egg donor who lived 600 miles away in order to minimize contact after the procedure was completed. We then had the task of creating an artificial menstrual cycle for Gita, so that the embryo would implant. We also had to coordinate Gita's cycle with that of the egg donor. Mark had completed his semen analysis—everything was normal, so we discussed steps to optimize his sperm function. I placed him on ConceptionXR, and we talked about him avoiding exposure to BioMutagens in his diet and while gardening, his favorite hobby. Gita was on a prenatal vitamin and a DHA supplement. I also encouraged her to add yoga to her fitness regimen of tennis, golf, and aerobics.

They flew the donor, a 25-year-old mother of two, and her husband to my office. She told me that she wanted to become an egg donor because she witnessed the anguish and difficulties a friend experienced while trying unsuccessfully to become pregnant. Over the next six weeks, the donor's ovaries were stimulated using BioIdentical FSH (Gonal-F) to promote egg development while she also used a BioAntagonist (Cetrotide) to prevent ovulation. Her response went very smoothly. Because the two women's cycles were synchronized, Gita's uterus would be ready for implantation when the embryo was ready. The egg retrieval yielded seven mature eggs. Mark provided a sperm specimen to the lab on the appointed day and fertilization took place in the lab. After five days, four of the oocytes had developed to the blastocyst stage. Mark and Gita elected to transfer one embryo and cryopreserve the others. Gita became pregnant and had a healthy baby girl. They still exchange greeting cards with their donor.

functional uterine factor and should either be treated with estradiol to help overcome the ovarian suppression or delay embryo transfer.

Consider an egg or embryo donor. Many fertility specialists, myself included, have a hard time admitting to patients that there's not much more we can do with their own eggs and sperm, and that they have to move on to the next level of treatment—using an egg or embryo donor. Aware of this tendency, I try to make sure that each patient has an honest and balanced assessment of her prognosis. Yet the statistics indicate that many women who go through ART don't get good counseling ahead of time or that they themselves are not ready to give up on their own genetic legacy.

But I encourage you to consider these statistics carefully: In 2004, of the more than 4,700 ART cycles performed on women over 43, only 8 percent resulted in a pregnancy and 4 percent actually had a live birth. In 2007, a review of nearly 300 cases performed on women between age 45 and 49 revealed a live birth rate of only 3.1 percent. None of the successful pregnancies was in a woman older than 45. By comparison, of women using donor eggs, the success rate for those 45 and older was 50 percent, and for women over 50, it was 40 percent.

I understand the desire most couples have to pass on their genes to the next generation. But while talking with women who are considering using a donor egg or donor embryo, I like to describe to them the indelible effect their own hormones, the food they eat, their level of stress, their level of calm, and practically everything else about their lifestyle while they're pregnant have upon any fetus that they carry. The hormones a fetus is exposed to in the womb have a direct and long-term impact on the baby's development—especially his brain development—his metabolism, and his personality. The bond created through this hormonal connection begins long before birth. Some of my patients find this information reassuring enough to feel more comfortable with their decision to consider working with an egg donor or adopting an embryo donated by another couple. In the end, you have to decide what's best for you.

Work with a gestational surrogate. Some women can't successfully complete a pregnancy, because they've had a hysterectomy or because of other medical problems. If, however, they have healthy ovaries, they can work with a gestational surrogate—a woman who carries and delivers the baby. This involves synchronizing your cycle with the surrogate's. Success rates have been very good with this technique. If you think you would consider a surrogate, talk to your fertility specialist, since many agencies have been set up to perform the necessary health screening and legal documents.

◆　◆　◆

I hope this introduction to ART has helped you to sort through the many treatment options. With this information, you should be able to make smart choices and better guide your treatment based on your fertility factors and your personal preferences. Your next step is to discuss your fertility factors, your fertility plan, your goals, and your concerns with your fertility specialist. In the conclusion of this book, I will discuss how to successfully navigate this potentially rough terrain.

Conclusion: Taking Action

A recent survey found that two-thirds to three-fourths of couples with infertility—including those with the best prognosis for success—do not pursue their goal of becoming parents because of a fear of failure. I think that's tragic. Many of the couples included in the survey assumed that they'd need the most expensive treatments, and that even these were rarely successful. This is completely untrue, and now you understand why—in many cases, less is more. Indeed, with the latest advances in fertility research, nearly 90 percent of those who wish to conceive and are willing to avail themselves of today's fertility treatments should be successful. Your fertility issues may not be so difficult to overcome.

My goal in writing this book is to show you that pregnancy may come easier to you than you think, simply by making lifestyle changes that improve your hormone balance. If you do need treatment, you don't necessarily need the barrage of diagnostic tests you'll be offered or the most advanced treatments to overcome your challenge. Morgan and I were able to become pregnant and have a child by using basic treatments combined with lifestyle changes that improved our hormone balance. Mostly, you should know that you have a choice, and the more knowledgeable you are the more you'll be able to exercise that choice.

Patients often feel overwhelmed when they enter the fertility world, and my hope is that this book has helped you to have a more positive experience.

By now, you have enough information to approach your decisions with confidence so that you can participate fully in the decision-making process. The last step is to choose a fertility center that's right for you and to learn to work with your specialists so you receive the most appropriate treatments at the lowest cost.

CHOOSING THE RIGHT CENTER

Most patients are not aware of the power that they have in choosing a center. Fertility centers are very competitive with one another and work hard to attract your attention. Since your goal is to find a specialist who will treat you as a partner in your health care, take some time to find the right person. Every center wants to attract the healthiest, most informed patients with the best possible prognosis—to boost the center's success rates. If you've gone through the Perfect Balance program, you likely fit this description. Also review this information if you've already been seen by someone but you're not sure that your treatment is going in the right direction.

Get a referral. One of the best ways to find a center is to ask other women or couples in your community whom they've seen and could recommend. You might be able to find these fertility patients through local branches of the national organizations like RESOLVE (www.resolve.org) and the American Fertility Association (www.theafa.org) or other local groups. Be sure to ask the people referring a provider about his ability to communicate and his willingness to discuss the diagnostic and treatment options. They should also feel that they were treated with respect, dignity, and kindness—key elements to keeping your stress hormones low. This character information is invaluable and should be at the top your list.

Check your specialist out. You're entitled to know the qualifications of your fertility specialist. Most specialists and centers are proud of their accomplishments and will include their credentials on their website. See if your physician is a member of ASRM (www.asrm.org)

and the Society for Reproductive Endocrinology and Infertility (www.socrei.org/SREImap.html). If the center's website doesn't provide this information, then call the office and ask for these specific credentials.

Check success rates. If a fertility center performs ART, it should be listed at the CDC website, http://apps.nccd.cdc.gov/ART2005/clinics05.usp or at http://www.sart.org/find_frm.html with an accurate posting of its most recently available success rate. Don't overinterpret the number. The best centers are the ones that attract the toughest patients, and therefore may have a lower success rate, whereas you can be misled by a mediocre center that will only select the easiest patients to treat and have a high success rate. Instead, look at how many cycles the center performs, what its multiple birth rates are (twins versus triplets and higher), and whether it has a large number of single embryo transfers, as well as the number of people it treats in your age range and with your types of issues. Don't dismiss a center because of these numbers, but be sure to discuss them during your consultation. If the center's specialists don't do ART procedures, ask them whom they will refer you to if it turns out that you'll need ART. Many reputable fertility specialists choose to free themselves of the overhead expenses by not maintaining their own equipment. But you'll want to be certain that they have an established relationship with a center that they're willing to stake their reputation on.

Confirm that the center can meet your needs. If you know that your options are severely limited, confirm ahead of time that it is equipped and prepared for whatever treatment you may need. Also, make sure a practitioner is available to see you on weekends or holidays. Ovulation does not always conveniently fall on a weekday, but that should not affect your treatment.

Inquire about financing. Many fertility centers offer financing plans that include a financial recovery (or refund) if you do not become pregnant. Just make certain that you don't forfeit the opportunity to perform a single or double embryo transfer in order to qualify for such deals—some may insist you use more embryos because using a larger number may increase your chance of a positive pregnancy test, but this would also increase your risk of pregnancy complications, including miscarriage. Many financing plans are very good deals, but just make sure that you read the fine print.

BE YOUR OWN ADVOCATE

When you see a fertility specialist, you'll likely find that you are rapidly categorized and placed on a protocol. There are endless combinations of variables from one couple to the next, so specialists tend to use this protocol approach based on the "average couple." But it is far from individualized. That's why it's up to you to guide your treatment center in how to best meet your needs.

Schedule a consultation. Get organized before your first appointment. If you're already being seen by a specialist, but want to rethink your treatment course, schedule a meeting for that purpose. Either way, plan to review everything that you've accomplished through this book—including the information on your preconception exams, the answers to your medical history questionnaires, and the chart on your fertility factors, including any diagnoses that have come out of your efforts to identify these factors. If the specialist is not familiar with suggestions in this book, offer to share the references with him. Today's standard is to practice *evidence-based medicine,* which means that as doctors, we update our treatments according to the latest research. The references in this book will reassure your specialist that my suggestions are valid unless there has been a more recent study to contradict this information. Don't feel like you'll offend the doctor by having an opinion and a plan. Many doctors respect patients for being educated health consumers and will welcome the opportunity to have intelligent discussions with them.

Be confident. Approach your consultation knowing that you've done everything you can—from balancing your hormones to learning about your fertility factors—to improve your chance of success. You should feel qualified to take an active role in the discussion and to communicate your ideas and preferences about the course of your treatment. Take notes so that you can remember what you discussed after you leave the appointment; it will also signal your doctor that you're on top of things and that she'll be held accountable for her recommendations.

Look for an out-of-the-box specialist. I spend a great deal of time traveling around the country lecturing to physicians. I try to educate them about the importance of underlying hormonal imbalance in treating patients and in improving fertility rates. I know that many physicians cling tightly to their current ways of practicing and are resistant to change. There is also a phenomenon within the fertility community that new technology is better. I totally agree that new technologies have opened doors to couples who would have otherwise been unable to bear children. But I also know that stepping back and looking at a person's overall health could provide more answers and raise success rates.

Check your fertility plan before and after any consultation appointment. Take notes so that you don't forget your key points or the answers that you receive. Review what you've done and what you're still willing to do. By taking these steps, you'll reach your goal as quickly as possible and also avoid repeating the same treatment over and over again without success.

Work as a team with your partner and you'll find that this process brings you together, rather than drives you apart. Though ART is thought of as being hard on couples, these high-tech treatments can be among the most empowering treatments imaginable, giving you back a sense of control over your life.

For many years, I have been privileged to help couples just like you plan their pregnancy, and I have been inspired by them to be a better partner in the patient-physician team. As a successful fertility patient myself, I've experienced firsthand the highs and lows of trying to have a baby. I know the journey can be frustrating and disappointing at times, but I always found hope in what I learned with each attempt at conception and with the many options that were available to us. I urge you to not give up, and to try to perceive each step you take, each attempt at conception, and each cycle of treatment as part of the journey that will get you closer to your goal of having a baby, rather than a series of false starts.

I know, based on the latest research and the success that my patients have experienced by following my hormone-balancing program, that many, many couples who are struggling with fertility issues can get pregnant if they balance their hormones and pursue some of the most basic steps to enhance their fertility. This should be comforting, but it does take a leap of faith. Your specialists might want you to rush forward to the most advanced treatments, but you may need to step back and take some time to get your bodies balanced first. This is never wasted time, because even if you do need more advanced treatments, your efforts to improve your lifestyle and your hormone balance will boost your success rates and get your pregnancy off to a healthy start. Our goal isn't a positive pregnancy test, but a healthy baby!

I hope this book has helped you to face any fears you have had, supported you in becoming your own advocate in your fertility treatment, and demonstrated that tuning in to your body, your symptoms, and each other are all important elements to successfully having a child with or without high-tech treatment.

APPENDIX A
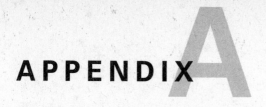

Use this calendar to record your menstrual flow and ovulation. Start on the first of each month. Record the days you spot with an "S" and the days of menstruation with an "L" for light, "M" for medium, and "H" for heavy. Write down the type of ovulation prediction kit you are using, and check the day when ovulation is detected and indicate the days around the time of ovulation that you and your partner are sexually active. Also keep track of other symptoms you are experiencing; these may serve as clues into your hormone balance. Use a value of 1 through 5, with 5 indicating the greatest severity. Make several copies of this chart and track your menstrual cycles for at least three months.

Day of Month	1	2	3	4	5	6	7	8	9	10	11	12	13	14	15	16	17	18	19	20	21	22	23	24	25	26	27	28	29	30	31
Menstrual flow																															
Ovulation detected/method used _____																															
Sexual activity																															
Stress level																															
Sleep disturbances																															
Pain (describe)																															
Constipation or diarrhea																															
Breast tenderness																															
Fatigue																															
Depression																															
Bloating																															
Vaginal mucus changes																															
Other:																															
Other:																															

APPENDIX B

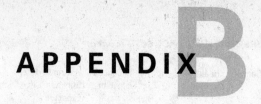

The following BioMutagens are commonly used and are known or strongly suspected to be a risk to your reproductive health, your fertility, your pregnancy, or the development of the fetus. Not all experts agree on the mode of action, the dose-toxicity relationship, and the health effects of BioMutagens but whenever scientific uncertainty exists, it's best to err on the side of caution. Try to minimize or avoid your exposure to the following BioMutagens by making careful choices about your diet and lifestyle. Any reduction in exposure will help.

BIOMUTAGENS IN PERSONAL CARE PRODUCTS

BioMutagen	Use and Source(s)	Health Concern for Him	Health Concern for Her	Health Concern for Embryo or Fetus	How to Avoid or Minimize Exposure
Phthalates	Used as a plasticizer in nail polish, nail treatment. Also used to extend the fragrance in scented products	Sperm DNA damage	Hormone disrupter	Adverse effect on the development of male reproductive organs	The majority of nail polish and nail treatments contain phthalates, so avoid them if possible. When choosing organic polishes, look for the word "phthalate" or "DBP," "DEP," or "DMP" on labels. If used as a fragrance, phthalates are rarely listed on labels; choose "fragrance-free" products.
Parabens	Widely used as preservatives in deodorants, shaving cream	Sperm damage Reduced sperm production	Hormone disrupter Possible carcinogen	Adverse effect on the development of male reproductive organs	Look for methyl-, ethyl-, propyl-, or butyl- parabens on labels.

(Cont'd)

BIOMUTAGENS IN PERSONAL CARE PRODUCTS *(Cont'd)*

BioMutagen	Use and Source(s)	Health Concern for Him	Health Concern for Her	Health Concern for Embryo or Fetus	How to Avoid or Minimize Exposure
Metals—lead acetate and mercury	Lead acetate can be found as a coloring in hair dye and some makeup, especially nonwestern cosmetics. Mercury may be used in small amounts as a preservative in eyedrops and artificial tears.	Carcinogen Neurotoxin	Hormone disrupter Carcinogen Neurotoxin	Possible link to autism and other brain development disorders	Read labels carefully. Avoid products containing the mercury compound "thimerosal."
Nonoxynol or nonylphenol ethoxylate	These petroleum-derived compounds are surfactants that make hair, skin, and facial products easier to disperse.	Hormone disrupters	Hormone disrupters	Birth defects	Read labels for these ingredients: polyethylene glycol (PEG) or the suffix "xynol," "cetareath," or "oleth."

BIOMUTAGENS IN FOODS AND COOKING

BioMutagen	Source(s)	Health Concern for Him	Health Concern for Her	Health Concern for Embryo or Fetus	What You Can Do to Avoid or Minimize Exposure
Mercury (methylmercury)	Contaminated fish or seafood	Sperm damage Decreased sperm production	Abnormal sperm motility Egg damage (to chromosomes)	Neurotoxicity Fetal brain damage	Restrict or eliminate tuna, swordfish, shark, king mackerel, tilefish, and grouper, as well as fish caught in any waters that are subject to a mercury advisory. When in doubt, avoid altogether.
Dioxin (TCDD) and dioxin-like compounds, polychlorinated dibenzofurans (PCDFs), and some polycholorinated biphenyls (PCBs)	Most exposure is from eating contaminated food, primarily high-fat foods such as meat, fish, and dairy products.	Reduced testosterone levels Hormone disrupters	Promotes endometriosis Hormone disrupters	Birth defects Developmental defects	Reduce dietary consumption of animal fats, fish, shellfish, and dairy products where dioxin accumulates.

BIOMUTAGENS IN FOODS AND COOKING (Cont'd)

BioMutagen	Source(s)	Health Concern for Him	Health Concern for Her	Health Concern for Embryo or Fetus	What You Can Do to Avoid or Minimize Exposure
Phthalates	Consumption of foods wrapped in clear food wraps, microwave cooking in certain plastics	Sperm DNA damage	Hormone disrupters	Adverse effect on the development of male reproductive organs	Use glass or ceramic containers to microwave food, don't allow plastic cling wrap to come into contact with hot or high-fat foods. Store food in glass, ceramic, or stainless steel. As a last resort use only #2, #4, or #5 plastics for food storage.
Bisphenol A (BPA)	The lining of many metal cans containing food and drink; and certain plastics in food and water containers and microwave ovenware. BPA migrates from liners into food and can leach from plastic containers.	Reduced sperm production Hormone disrupters	Miscarriage Hormone disrupters	Adverse effect on the development of male reproductive organs	Hand wash plastic dishware with mild soap in warm—not hot—water. Discard plastic that is cracked or that appears cloudy. Switch to #5 polypropylene bottles. Purchase soups packaged in cardboard cartons and beans and vegetables in glass jars when available.
Pesticides	Consumption of conventionally grown fruits and vegetables	Reduced sperm production Sperm damage Hormone disrupter	Miscarriage Hormone disrupters Menstrual irregularities	Birth defects Growth retardation Adverse effect on the development of reproductive tract (primarily male)	Choose organic produce when possible. Otherwise wash and rinse to reduce your exposure.
Alcohol	Alcoholic beverages	Decreased libido Reduced sperm quality	Decreased libido Ovulatory dysfunction Reduced implantation	Fetal alcohol syndrome Miscarriage	Avoid alcohol while attempting to conceive.

(Cont'd)

BIOMUTAGENS IN FOODS AND COOKING (Cont'd)

BioMutagen	Source(s)	Health Concern for Him	Health Concern for Her	Health Concern for Embryo or Fetus	What You Can Do to Avoid or Minimize Exposure
Carbon monoxide, nicotine, and cotinine	Tobacco smoke— first and secondhand	Reduced sperm count Reduced sperm motility Carcinogenic	Accelerated ovarian aging Decreased uterine blood flow	Growth retardation	Implement a plan to stop smoking as soon as possible. Talk to your doctor if you think you need assistance.

BIOMUTAGENS AT HOME

BioMutagen	Use/Source(s)	Health Concern for Him	Health Concern for Her	Health Concern for Embryo or Fetus	What You Can Do to Avoid or Minimize Exposure
Phthalates	These widely used industrial plasticizers give flexibility to shower curtains, vinyl products such as wall covering and flooring and fake leather, and add resilience to polyvinyl chloride (PVC) products, as well as new auto interiors.	Sperm DNA damage	Hormone disrupters	Adverse effect on the development of male reproductive organs	When possible, choose alternatives to vinyl products, replace PVC plastics with phthalate-free plastic or hard plastic alternatives. Try to air out products with a "plastic" odor for several days to vaporize the phthalates.
Polybrominated diphenyl ethers (PBDEs)	Flame retardants in furniture foam padding, carpet padding, and electronics	Reduced sperm production	Safety unknown	Altered brain development	Replace or cover furniture with exposed foam. Use care when replacing the carpet pad; avoid contact if possible. Purchase products from manufacturers that use alternatives to PBDEs.

BIOMUTAGENS AT HOME (Cont'd)

BioMutagen	Use/Source(s)	Health Concern for Him	Health Concern for Her	Health Concern for Embryo or Fetus	What You Can Do to Avoid or Minimize Exposure
Perfluoro-chemicals (PFCs)	Industrial chemicals widely used as flame retardants and stain, water, and grease repellents	Hormone disrupters	Hormone disrupters	Safety unknown	Avoid treated furniture, clothing, and food wrap. Teflon and Scotchgard are commonly used products to avoid.
Chlorine, benzene, alkylphenoxyl ethanols	Common ingredients in household cleaning products	Hormone disrupters	Hormone disrupters	Birth defects	Select nontoxic alternatives such as Seventh Generation or Bio-Kleen.
Organophos-phorous insecticide (e.g. acephate, dichlorvos, dimethoate, disulfoton, malathion, naled, phosmet, tetrachlorvinphos and trichlorfon, methyl parathion, chlorpyrifos-methyl)	Pesticides, insecticides	Reduced sperm production Increased percentage of abnormal sperm Possible carcinogen	Alteration of menstrual cycles Accelerated loss of eggs	Increased incidence of miscarriage	To avoid use of exterminating products, bugproof your house. Tightly seal food and beverage containers, seal entryways, dust with boric acid on cracks and crevices outdoors, try bait boxes or fatty acid soaps, hire an integrated pest management (IPM) expert.

BIOMUTAGENS IN THE WORKPLACE

BioMutagen	Use/Source(s)	Health Concern for Him	Health Concern for Her	Health Concern for Embryo or Fetus	What You Can Do to Avoid or Minimize Exposure
Toluene, benzene, xylene—common volatile and semivolatile organic compounds (VOCs) (SVOCs)	Common chemical solvents found in the textile and painting industries, plastic ink and dye manufacturing plants, and from fuel	Reduced sperm motility Hormone disrupters	Hormone disrupters	Impaired fetal development Birth defects	Review all material safety data sheets (MSDSs), ventilate area whenever possible or use appropriate protective gear. Wash hands before eating or drinking.

(Cont'd)

BIOMUTAGENS IN THE WORKPLACE *(Cont'd)*

BioMutagen	Use/Source(s)	Health Concern for Him	Health Concern for Her	Health Concern for Embryo or Fetus	What You Can Do to Avoid or Minimize Exposure
Glycol ethers	Industrial organic solvents found as a coating in paints, thinner, dyes, inks, varnish, and semiconductor chips, as cleaners and degreasers in dry-cleaning and circuit board manufacture, and as an additive to brake fluid, jet fuel, and deicing solutions	Testicular atrophy Diminished sperm count	Reduced implantation	Birth defects Increased risk of low birth weight Increased risk of miscarriage	Use in a well-ventilated area or with a respirator. Use personal protective equipment, review all MSDSs, prevent exposure, or request a transfer. Wash hands before eating or drinking. Use the less harmful water-based paints when possible.
Chemo-therapeutic agents	Cancer treatment	Lowered sperm count Reduced sperm motility	Reduced implantation Accelerated loss of eggs Menstrual irregularities	Birth defects Increased risk of miscarriage	Use personal protective equipment and avoid mixing or administering whenever possible. Wash hands before eating or drinking when handling toxic agents.
Pesticides, insecticides	Chemical agents widely used by farmers, landscapers, gardeners, and exterminators	Lowered sperm count	Reduced implantation Menstrual irregularity	Miscarriage	Use personal protective equipment and avoid skin and eye contact. Wash hands before eating or drinking. Keep work clothes separate from general laundry.

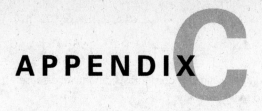

APPENDIX C

Use these guidelines to determine the level of care you need, and the qualifications you should look for in an expert, based on your individual situation.

Level 1 Care (basic fertility issues)

Patient Inclusion Criteria
- The duration of the infertility is less than 24 months.
- The female partner is less than 30 years of age.
- There are no risk factors for pelvic disease or male reproductive abnormalities.
- The couple has undergone less than 4 months of treatment without success.

Practitioner Qualifications
- Is knowledgeable about the prerequisites for successful reproduction.
- Is prepared to consult, educate, and advise both partners.

Responsibility
- Interview and physical examination.
- Confirmation of ovulation.
- Interpretation of semen analysis.
- Timely referral of patients who exceed Level 1 criteria or have complex disorders.

Level 2 Care (moderate fertility issues)

Patient Inclusion Criteria
- The duration of the infertility is less than 36 months.
- The female partner is less than 35 years of age.
- The couple does not qualify for Level 1 care.

Practitioner Qualifications
- Possesses all qualifications for Level 1 care.
- Possesses certification or documented experience in the necessary endocrinologic, gynecologic, or urologic procedures.
- Is knowledgeable about the effectiveness, adverse effects, and costs of the diagnosis and current treatment of infertility.

*Modified from Guidelines for the Provision of Infertility Services, 1996, ASRM.

Responsibility

- Assessment of tubal patency.
- Management of uncomplicated anovulation, endometriosis, and tubal disease.
- Management of uncomplicated male infertility.
- Access to necessary laboratory services seven days a week during treatment.
- Available for cycle management seven days per week during treatment.
- Timely referral of patients who exceed Level 2 criteria or have complex disorders.

Level 3 Care (complex fertility issues)

Patient Inclusion Criteria

- The couple does not qualify for Level 1 or 2 care.
- Assisted reproductive technology (ART) is under consideration

Practitioner Qualifications

- Possesses all qualifications for Level 1 and Level 2 care.
- Possesses certification or documented experience in reproductive endocrinology, urology/andrology or assisted reproductive technology.
- Ability to provide access to counseling services

Responsibility

- Management of complicated anovulation, endometriosis, and tubal disease.
- Management of complicated male infertility.
- Able to provide access to male and female microsurgical services, and ART and related services

APPENDIX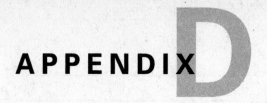

Use this fertility plan to record your preferences in case you decide to pursue fertility treatment. It's helpful to try to answer these questions before you start treatment, as your preferences will influence which treatment options you choose. Write down any feelings or explanations surrounding these issues. Work together with your partner so that you're both in agreement. If you find that you can't agree on an issue, come back to it later, perhaps after you've had a bit of experience with fertility treatments. You can always come back to your plan to revise or complete it as your feelings evolve. One note: Many of the terms are covered in the final treatment section of this book—chapters 13 and 14.

How many children do you wish to have? _____

Ideally, how many years would you like between your children?

_____

_____

How do you feel about the following kinds of fertility treatment?

• Ovulation induction

_____

_____

• Insemination

_____

_____

• IVF

_____

_____

• Assisted hatching

_____

_____

◆ ICSI (sperm implantation)

_____

_____

Is there any kind of treatment you and your partner will not consider?

_____

_____

How do you and your partner feel about using donated sperm?

_____

_____

How do you and your partner feel about using donated embryos?

_____

_____

How do you and your partner feel about having twins?

_____

_____

What about having triplets or higher-order multiple gestation pregnancies?

_____

_____

Would you and your partner consider selective reduction if you became
pregnant with triplets or a higher-order multiple pregnancy?

_____

_____

Would you and your partner consider adopting a child?

_____

_____

How do you and your partner feel about freezing extra embryos for a later
pregnancy?

_____

_____

Would you and your partner consider donating extra embryos to other couples seeking fertility treatment or for stem cell research?

_____

_____

Are you and your partner interested in testing to see if either of you are carriers for any inheritable diseases?

_____

_____

Do you and your partner want to know the sex of your baby before birth?

_____

_____

What method of postpartum birth control are you planning?

_____

_____

Do you and your partner have any fears related to fertility treatment or pregnancy that haven't been addressed here?

_____

_____

APPENDIX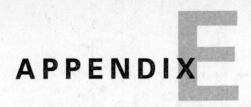

FITNESS JOURNAL

Use this as a template for a fitness journal. Enter your fitness and weight goals at the beginning of the journal, and each week enter your weight and resting heart rate as well as the number of minutes you exercise each day. To measure your resting heart rate, take your pulse for 60 seconds before you get out of bed in the morning.

Fitness goal in three months: _____

Weight goal in three months: _____

EXERCISE LOG

Week of _____ Weight _____ Resting Heart Rate _____

(Aim for 40- to 60-minute sessions every day, but don't beat yourself up if you fall short of this goal.)

	M	T	W	Th	F	Sat	Sun
Walking/aerobic exercise							
Yoga/stretching							
Strength training							

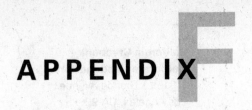

APPENDIX F

Dr. Robert Greene
Sher Institute for Reproductive
Medicine
2288 Auburn Blvd, Suite 204
Sacramento, CA 95821
Phone: 877-263-4040
www.RobertGreeneMD.com
www.Haveababy.com

**American Society for
Reproductive Medicine**
1209 Montgomery Highway
Birmingham, Alabama
35216-2809
Phone: 205-978-5000
Fax: 205-978-5005
www.asrm.org

**Society for Reproductive
Endocrinologists**
1209 Montgomery Highway
Birmingham, AL 35216-2809
Phone: 205-978-5000
Fax: 205-978-5005
www.socrei.org

**Centers for Disease Control
and Prevention
CDC/DRH**
4770 Buford Hwy, NE
MS K-20
Atlanta, GA 30341-3717
Phone: 770-488-5200
www.cdc.gov/art

**Society for Assisted
Reproductive Technology**
1209 Montgomery Highway
Birmingham, AL 35216
Phone: 205-978-5000
Fax: 205-978-5015
www.sart.org

RESOLVE
7910 Woodmont Avenue,
Suite 1350
Bethesda, MD 20814
Phone: 301-652-8585
Fax: 301-652-9375
www.resolve.org

American Fertility Association
305 Madison Avenue, Suite 449
New York, NY 10165
Phone: 888-917-3777
www.theafa.org

Fertile Hope
65 Broadway, Suite 603
New York, NY 10006
Phone: 888-994-HOPE
www.fertilehope.org

Fertility LifeLines
Phone: 866-538-7879
www.fertilitylifelines.com

The InterNational Council on Infertility Information Dissemination
PO Box 6836
Arlington, VA 22206
Phone: 703-379-9178
Fax: 703-379-1593
www.inciid.com

Endometriosis Association
8585 N. 76th Place
Milwaukee, WI 53223 USA
Phone: 414-355-2200
Fax: 414-355-6065
www.endometriosisassn.org

Polycystic Ovarian Syndrome Association
PO Box 3403
Englewood, CO 80111
www.pcosupport.org

Turner Syndrome Society of the United States
14450 TC Jester, Suite 260
Houston TX 77014
Toll Free: 800-365-9944
Phone: 832-249-9988
Fax: 832-249-9987
www.turner-syndrome-us.org

Polycystic Ovarian Syndrome Association
PO Box 3403
Englewood, CO 80111
Phone: 877-775-PCOS
www.pcosupport.org

California Cryobank Corporate Headquarters
11915 La Grange Avenue
Los Angeles, CA 90025
Phone: 310-443-5244
Fax: 310-443-5258
Toll Free: 800-977-3761
www.cryobank.com

Men's Health Network
P.O. Box 75972
Washington, DC 20013
Phone: 202-543-6461
www.menshealthnetwork.org

Union of Concerned Scientists National Headquarters
2 Brattle Square
Cambridge, MA 02238-9105
Phone: 617-547-5552
Fax: 617-864-9405
www.ucsusa.org

Campaign for Safe Cosmetics
Info@safecosmetics.org
www.safecosmetics.org

Environmental Working Group Headquarters
1436 U St. NW, Suite 100
Washington, DC 20009
Phone: 202-667-6982
www.ewg.org
www.cosmeticdatabase.com

Organic Consumers Association
6771 South Silver Hill Drive
Finland, MN 55603
Phone: 218-226-4164
Fax: 218-353-7652
www.organicconsumers.org

ConsumerLab.com, LLC
333 Mamaroneck Avenue
White Plains, NY 10605
Phone: 914-722-9149
www.consumerlab.com

Chemical Body Burden
PO Box 8743
Missoula, MT 59807
www.chemicalbodyburden.org

**Pesticide Action Network
North America**
49 Powell St., Suite 500
San Francisco, CA 94102
Phone: 415-981-1771
www.panna.org

**Center for Science in the
Public Interest**
1875 Connecticut Ave. NW
Suite 300
Washington, DC 20009
Phone: 202-332-9110
Fax: 202-265-4954
www.cspinet.org

Food News
1436 U Street NW, Suite 100
Washington, DC 20009
Phone: 212-667-6982
www.foodnews.org

REFERENCES

Author's note: The publications listed here do not represent an exhaustive list of those cited throughout the book. In the field of medicine, information is always evolving as new studies become available. As a result, it is difficult for many health care providers to remain up to date on this subject unless they make a special effort to do so. The papers listed here are those that could have easily been overlooked or those that might have needed a citation because, without full knowledge of the research, they might seem controversial. I encourage you to use this list to introduce discussion with your health care provider about any of the information contained in this book.

Chapter 1 ◆ Hormone Balance: The Foundation of Fertility

Ebling, F. J. P. (2005). "The neuroendocrine timing of puberty." *Reproduction* **129**(6): 675–683.

Greene, R., and L. Feldon (2005). *Dr. Robert Greene's Perfect Balance*. Three Rivers Press, New York.

Kapoor, D., and T. H. Jones (2005). "Smoking and hormones in health and endocrine disorders." *Eur J Endocrinol* **152**(4): 491–499.

Nohr, E. A., B. H. Bech, et al. (2005). "Prepregnancy obesity and fetal death: A study within the Danish national birth cohort." *Obstet Gynecol* **106**(2): 250–259.

Tarin, J. J., and V. Gomez-Piquer (2002). "Do women have a hidden heat period?" *Hum Reprod* **17**(9): 2243–2248.

Chapter 2 ◆ Protecting Your Fertility

Farr, S., J. Cai, et al. (2006). "Pesticide exposure and timing of menopause. The Agricultural Health Study." *Amer Epidemiol* **163**: 731–742.

Federman, D. D. (2006). "The biology of human sex differences." *N Engl J Med* **354**(14): 1507–14.

Genuis, S. J. (2006). "Health issues and the environment—an emerging paradigm for providers of obstetrical and gynaecological health care." *Hum Reprod* **21**(9): 2201–2208.

Gosden, R. G., and A. P. Feinberg (2007). "Genetics and epigenetics—nature's pen-and-pencil set." *N Engl J Med* **356**(7): 731–733.

Grandjean, P. and P. Landrigan (2006). "Developmental neurotoxicity of industrial chemicals." *Lancet* **368:** 2167–2178.

Kleinhaus, K., M. Perrin, et al. (2006). "Paternal age and spontaneous abortion." *Obstet Gynecol* **108**(2): 369–377.

Kline, J., A. Kinney, et al. (2005). "Predictors of antral follicle count during the reproductive years." *Hum Reprod:* **20**(8): 2179–2189.

Ramsay, J. E., I. Greer, et al. (2006). "Obesity and reproduction." *BMJ* **333**(7579): 1159–1162.

Rizzolio, F., S. Bione, et al. (2006). "Chromosomal rearrangements in Xq and premature ovarian failure: Mapping of 25 new cases and review of the literature." *Hum Reprod* **21**(6): 1477–1483.

Ross, M., D. Grafham, et al. (2005). "The DNA sequence of the human X chromosome." *Nature* **434:** 325–337.

Simon, B., S. J. Lee, et al. (2005). "Preserving fertility after cancer." *CA Cancer J Clin* **55**(4): 211–228.

Swales, A. K. E., and N. Spears (2005). "Genomic imprinting and reproduction." *Reproduction* **130**(4): 389–399.

Chapter 3 ◆ Preconception Planning

—. "Smoking and infertility." *Fertil and Steril* **86**(5) (2006): S172–S177.

—. "Status of environmental and dietary estrogens—are they significant estrogens?" *Fertil and Steril* **86**(5) (2006): S218–S220.

—. "Vaccination guidelines for female infertility patients." *Fertil and Steril* **86**(5) (2006): S28–S30.

Evans, J. (2006). "Pregnancy appears to be safe after recent bariatric surgery." *OB Gyn News:* 10.

Seibel, M. (2006). "The environment: Its risks to conception and pregnancy." *Sexual, Reprod & Menopause* **4**(1): 1–2.

Wiegratz, J. R., et al. (2006). "Fertility after discontinuation of treatment with an oral contraceptive containing 30 mg of ethinyl estradiol and 2 mg of dienogest." *Fertil and Steril* **85**(6): 1812–1819.

Chapter 4 ◆ Eating Right for Fertility

Agarwal, A., S. A. Prabakaran, et al. (2005). "Prevention of oxidative stress injury to sperm." *J Androl* **26**(6): 654–660.

Ahuja, K. D. K., I. K. Robertson, et al. (2006). "Effects of chili consumption on postprandial glucose, insulin, and energy metabolism." *Am J Clin Nutr* **84**(1): 63–69.

Anway, M. D. and M. K. Skinner (2006). "Epigenetic transgenerational actions of endocrine disruptors." *Endocrinology* **147**(6): s43–49.

Balercia, R., et al. (2005). "Placebo-controlled double-blind randomized trial on the use of l-carnitine, l-acetylcarnitine, or combined l-carnitine and l-acetylcarnitine in men with idiopathic asthenozoospermia." *Fertil and Steril* **84**(3): 662–671.

Berkow, S., and N. Bernard (2006). "Vegetarian diets and weight status." *Nutrit Rev* **64**(4): 175–188.

Bodnar, L. M., G. Tang, et al. (2006). "Periconceptional multivitamin use reduces the risk of preeclampsia." *Am J Epidemiol* **164**(5): 470–477.

Budak, E., M. Sanchez, et al. (2006). "Interactions of the hormones leptin, ghrelin, adiponectin, resistin and PYY3-36 with the reproductive system." *Fertil & Steril* **85**(6): 1563–1581.

Chia, S. E., C. N. Ong, et al. (2000). "Comparison of zinc concentrations in blood and seminal plasma and the various sperm parameters between fertile and infertile men." *J Androl* **21**(1): 53–57.

Devereux, G., S. W. Turner, et al. (2006). "Low maternal vitamin E intake during pregnancy is associated with asthma in 5-year-old children." *Am J Respir Crit Care Med* **174**(5): 499–507.

Eskenazi, B., S. A. Kidd, et al. (2005). "Antioxidant intake is associated with semen quality in healthy men." *Hum Reprod* **20**(4): 1006–1012.

Farr, S. L., G. S. Cooper, et al. (2004). "Pesticide use and menstrual cycle characteristics among premenopausal women in the agricultural health study." *Am J Epidemiol* **160**(12): 1194–1204.

Garland, C. F., et al. (2006). "The role of vitamin D in cancer prevention." *Am J Public Health* **96**(2): 252–261.

Gartner, R., B. C. H. Gasnier, et al. (2002). "Selenium supplementation in patients with autoimmune thyroiditis decreases thyroid peroxidase antibodies concentrations." *J Clin Endocrinol Metab* **87**(4): 1687–1691.

Group, E. C. W. (2006). "Nutrition and reproduction in women." *Hum Reprod Update* **12**(3): 193–207.

Hawkes, W. C., and N. L. Keim (2003). "Dietary selenium intake modulates thyroid hormone and energy metabolism in men." *J Nutr* **133**(11): 3443–3448.

Hawkes, W. C. and P. J. Turek (2001). "Effects of dietary selenium on sperm motility in healthy men." *J Androl* **22**(5): 764–772.

He, K., K. Liu, et al. (2006). "Magnesium intake and incidence of metabolic syndrome among young adults." *Circulation* **113**(13): 1675–1682.

Hill, P. B., L. Garbaczewski, et al. (1986). "Gonadotrophin release and meat consumption in vegetarian women." *Am J Clin Nutr* **43**(1): 37–41.

Hollowell, J. G., N. W. Staehling, et al. (1998). "Iodine nutrition in the United States. Trends and public health implications: Iodine excretion data from National Health and Nutrition Examination Surveys I and III (1971–1974 and 1988–1994)." *J Clin Endocrinol Metab* **83**(10): 3401–3408.

Johnston, C. S. (2005). "Strategies for healthy weight loss: From vitamin C to the glycemic response." *J Am Coll Nutr* **24**(3): 158–165.

Julian, D., and C. Leeuwenburgh (2004). "Linkage between insulin and the free radical theory of aging." *Am J Physiol Regul Integr Comp Physiol* **286**(1): R20–21.

Kiefer, I., T. Rathmanner, et al. (2005). "Eating and dieting differences in men and women." *Men's Health and Gender* **2**(2): 186–193.

Lenzi, A., F. Lombardo, et al. (2003). "Use of carnitine therapy in selected cases of male factor infertility: a double-blind crossover trial." *Fertil and Steril* **79**(2): 292–300.

Lydic, McNurlan, et al. (2006). "Chromium picolinate improves insulin sensitivity in obese subjects with polycystic ovary syndrome." *Fertil and Steril* **86**(1): 243–246.

Mori, A., S. Lehmann, et al. (2006). "Capsaicin, a component of red peppers, inhibits the growth of androgen-independent, p53 mutant prostate cancer cells." *Cancer Res* **66**(6): 3222–3229.

Ng, C. M., M. R. Blackman, et al. (2004). "The role of carnitine in the male reproductive system." *Ann NY Acad Sci* **1033**(1): 177–188.

Oltmanns, K. M., B. Fruehwald-Schultes, et al. (2001). "Hypoglycemia, but not insulin, acutely decreases LH and T secretion in men." *J Clin Endocrinol Metab* **86**(10): 4913–4919.

Pasquali, R. (2006). "Obesity, fat distribution and infertility." *Maturitas* **54**: 363–371.

Pocar, P., T. A. Brevini, et al. (2003). "The impact of endocrine disruptors on oocyte competence." *Reproduction* **125**(3): 313–325.

Scherer, P. E. (2006). "Adipose tissue: From lipid storage compartment to endocrine organ." *Diabetes* **55**(6): 1537–1545.

Sewell, P. Huston, et al. (2006). "Increased neonatal fat mass, not lean body mass, is associated with maternal obesity." *Ameri J Obstet and Gyn* **195**(4): 1100–1103.

Steinman, G. (2006). "Mechanisms of twinning: VII. Effect of diet and heredity on the human twinning rate." *J Reprod Med* **51**(5): 405–410.

Turker, O., K. Kumanlioglu, et al. (2006). "Selenium treatment in autoimmune thyroiditis: 9-month follow-up with variable doses." *J Endocrinol* **190**(1): 151–156.

Vega, G. L., B. Adams-Huet, et al. (2006). "Influence of body fat content and distribution on variation in metabolic risk." *J Clin Endocrinol Metab* **91**(11): 4459–4466.

Wade, G., and J. Jones (2004). "Neuroendocrinology of nutritional infertility." *Amer J Physiol* **287**: R1277–1296.

Wong, W. Y., H. M. W. M. Merkus, et al. (2002). "Effects of folic acid and zinc sulfate on male factor subfertility: A double-blind, randomized, placebo-controlled trial." *Fertil and Steril* **77**(3): 491–498.

Wu, Y., W. G. Foster, et al. (2006). "Rapid effects of pesticides on human granulosa-lutein cells." *Reproduction* **131**(2): 299–310.

Zhang, C., S. Liu, et al. (2006). "Dietary fiber intake, dietary glycemic load, and the risk for gestational diabetes mellitus." *Diabet Care* **29**(10): 2223–2230.

Chapter 5 ◆ Shaping Up to Promote Pregnancy

Gerstein, H. C., and L. Waltman (2006). "Why don't pigs get diabetes? Explanations for variations in diabetes susceptibility in human populations living in a diabetogenic environment." *CMAJ* **174**(1): 25–26.

Jonge, J. D. (2003). "Effects of the menstrual cycle on exercise performance." *Sports Med* **33**(11): 833–851.

Kumru, H., R. Ozmerdivenli, et al. (2005). "Effects of regular physical exercise on serum leptin and androgen concentrations in young women." *Men's Health and Gen* **2**(2): 218–222.

Levine, J. A., L. M. Lanningham-Foster, et al. (2005). "Interindividual variation in posture allocation: Possible role in human obesity." *Science* **307**(5709): 584–586.

Morris, S. N., S. A. Missmer, et al. (2006). "Effects of lifetime exercise on the outcome of in vitro fertilization." *Obstet Gynecol* **108**(4): 938–945.

Nabkasorn, C., N. Miyai, et al. (2006). "Effects of physical exercise on depression, neuroendocrine stress hormones and physiological fitness in adolescent females with depressive symptoms." *Eur J Public Health* **16**(2): 179–184.

Nicklas, B. J., T. You, et al. (2005). "Behavioural treatments for chronic systemic inflammation: Effects of dietary weight loss and exercise training." *CMAJ* **172**(9): 1199–1209.

Shadid, S., C. D. A. Stehouwer, et al. (2006). "Diet/exercise versus pioglitazone: Effects of insulin sensitization with decreasing or increasing fat mass on adipokines and inflammatory markers." *J Clin Endocrinol Metab* **91**(9): 3418–3425.

Southorn, T. (2002). "Great balls of fire and the vicious cycle: A study of the effects of cycling on male fertility." *J Fam Plan and Reprod Health Care* **28**(4): 211–213.

Wallis, G. A., R. Dawson, et al. (2006). "Metabolic response to carbohydrate ingestion during exercise in males and females." *Am J Physiol Endocrinol Metab* **290**(4): E708–715.

Warburton, D. E. R., C. W. Nicol, et al. (2006). "Health benefits of physical activity: The evidence." *CMAJ* **174**(6): 801–809.

Warburton, D. E. R., C. W. Nicol, et al. (2006). "Prescribing exercise as preventive therapy." *CMAJ* **174**(7): 961–974.

Warren, M. P., and N. E. Perlroth (2001). "The effects of intense exercise on the female reproductive system." *J Endocrinol* **170**(1): 3–11.

Wee, S. L., C. Williams, et al. (2005). "Ingestion of a high-glycemic index meal increases muscle glycogen storage at rest but augments its utilization during subsequent exercise." *J Appl Physiol* **99**(2): 707–714.

Chapter 6 ◆ Coping with Stress to Boost Fertility

—. (2005). "The stress and distress of infertility: Does religion help women cope?" *Sexual, Reprod & Menopause* **3**(2): 45–51.

Bethea, Pau, et al. (2005). "Sensitivity to stress-induced reproductive dysfunction linked to activity of the serotonin system." *Fertil and Steril* **83**(1): 148–155.

Breen, K. M., H. J. Billings, et al. (2005). "Endocrine basis for disruptive effects of cortisol on preovulatory events." *Endocrinol* **146**(4): 2107–2115.

Bjornerem, A., B. Straume, et al. (2006). "Seasonal variation of estradiol, follicle-stimulating hormone, and dehydroepiandrosterone sulfate in women and men." *J Clin Endocrinol Metab* **91**(10): 3798–3802.

Boden, M. J., and D. J. Kennaway (2006). "Circadian rhythms and reproduction." *Reproduction* **132**(3): 379–392.

Boivin, J., and L. Schmidt (2005). "Infertility-related stress in men and women predicts treatment outcome 1 year later." *Fertil and Steril* **83**(6): 1745–1752.

Grewen, K. M., S. S. Girdler, et al. (2005). "Effects of partner support on resting oxytocin, cortisol, norepinephrine, and blood pressure before and after warm partner contact." *Psychosom Med* **67**(4): 531–538.

Harrison, R. F. (1988). "Stress spikes of hyperprolactinaemia and infertility." *Hum Reprod* **3**(2): 173–175.

Lazar, S., G. Bush, et al. (2000). "Functional brain mapping of the relaxation response and meditation." *NeuroReport* **11**(7): 1581–1585.

Peterson, B. D., C. R. Newton, et al. (2006). "Gender differences in how men and women who are referred for IVF cope with infertility stress." *Hum Reprod* **21**(9): 2443–2449.

Pook, M., W. Krause, et al. (1999). "Coping with infertility: Distress and changes in sperm quality." *Hum Reprod* **14**(6): 1487–1492.

Schmidt, L., B. E. Holstein, et al. (2005). "Communication and coping as predictors of fertility problem stress: Cohort study of 816 participants who did not achieve a delivery after 12 months of fertility treatment." *Hum Reprod* **20**(11): 3248–3256.

Williams, N. I., S. Berga, et al. (2007). "Synergism between psychosocial and metabolic stressors: Impact upon reproductive function in cynomolgus monkeys." *Am J Physiol Endocrinol Metab* **293**(1): E 270–276.

Younglai, E. V., A. C. Holloway, et al. (2005). "Environmental and occupational factors affecting fertility and IVF success." *Hum Reprod Update* **11**(1): 43–57.

Chapter 7 ◆ Your First Steps to Pregnancy Start at Home

Agarwal, S., et al. (2005). "Changes in sperm motility and chromatin integrity following contact with vaginal lubricants." *Fertil and Steril* **84:** S73–S73.

Bjorndahl, L., J. Kirkman-Brown, et al. (2006). "Development of a novel home sperm test." *Hum Reprod* **21**(1): 145–149.

Conde-Agudelo, A., A. Rosa-Bermudez, et al. (2006). "Birth spacing and risk of adverse perinatal outcomes: A meta-analysis." *JAMA* **295**(15): 1809–1823.

Cousineau, T., T. Green, et al. (2006). "Development and validation of the infertility self-efficacy scale." *Fertil and Steril* **85**(6): 1684–1696.

Dunn, K., L. Cherkas, et al. (2005). "Genetic influences on variation in female orgasmic function: A twin study." *Biol Letters* **1**(3): 260–263.

Ellington, J., and J. Schimmels (2004). "The effects of vaginal lubricants and moisturizers on computer assisted sperm analysis (CASA) parameters associated with cervical mucus penetration." *Fertil and Steril* **82**: S145–S146.

Ellington, J., Daugherty, et al. (2003). "Prevalence of vaginal dryness in trying-to-conceive couples." *Fertil and Steril* **79**: 21–22.

Gesink Law, D. C., R. F. Maclehose, et al. (2007). "Obesity and time to pregnancy." *Hum Reprod* **22**(2): 414–420.

Gleicher, N., and D. Barad (2006). "Unexplained infertility: Does it really exist?" *Hum Reprod* **21**(8): 1951–1955.

Modest, G. A., and J. J. W. Fangman (2002). "Nipple piercing and hyperprolactinemia." *N Engl J Med* **347**(20): 1626–1627.

O'Connor, K. A., E. Brindle, et al. (2006). "Ovulation detection methods for urinary hormones: Precision, daily and intermittent sampling and a combined hierarchical method." *Hum Reprod* **21**(6): 1442–1452.

Robinson, J., M. Wakelin, et al. (2007). "Increased pregnancy rate with use of the Clearblue Easy Fertility Monitor." Unipath Ltd., Bedford, United Kingdom." *Fertil and Steril* **87**(2): 329–334.

Samuels, M. H., K. G. Schuff, et al. (2007). "Health status, mood and cognition in experimentally induced subclinical hypothyroidism." *J Clin Endocrinol Metab* **92**(7): 2545–2551.

Sievert, L., and C. Dubois (2005). "Validating signals of ovulation: Do women who think they know, really know?" *Am J Hum Biol* **17**(3): 310–320.

Trokoudes, K., N. Skordi, et al. (2006). "Infertility and thyroid disease." *Curr Opin Obstet Gynecol* **18**: 446–451.

Waller, D. K., A. M. Sweeney, et al. (1996). "Pregnancy and the timing of intercourse." *N Engl J Med* **334**(19): 1266–1268.

Wilcox, A., C. Weinberg, et al. (1995). "Timing of sexual intercourse in relation to ovulation." *N Engl J Med* **333**(23): 1517–1521.

Wilcox, A. J., D. D. Baird, et al. (1999). "Time of implantation of the conceptus and loss of pregnancy." *N Engl J Med* **340**(23): 1796–1799.

Chapter 8 ◆ Male Factor

—. (2006). "The clinical utility of sperm DNA integrity testing." *Fertil and Steril* **86**(5): S35–S37.

—. (2006). "Report on evaluation of the azoospermic male." *Fertil and Steril* **86**(5): S210–S215.

—. (2006). "Report on optimal evaluation of the infertile male." *Fertil and Steril* **86**(5): S202–S209.

—. (2006). "Report on varicocele and infertility." *Fertil and Steril* **86**(5): S93–S95.

—. (2006). "Treatment of androgen deficiency in the aging male." *Fertil and Steril* **86**(5): S236–S240.

Auger, J., J. M. Kunstmann, et al. (1995). "Decline in semen quality among fertile men in Paris during the past 20 years." *N Engl J Med* **332**(5): 281–285.

Bhasin, S. (2007). "Approach to the infertile man." *J Clin Endocrinol Metab* **92**(6): 1995–2004.

Boschert, S. (2002). "Air pollution may impair sperm number, quality." *Ob Gyn News* **37**(13): 21.

Carlsen, E., J. H. Petersen, et al. (2004). "Effects of ejaculatory frequency and season on variations in semen quality." *Fertil and Steril* **82**(2): 358–366.

Claman, P. (2004). "Men at risk: Occupation and male infertility." *Fertil and Steril* **81:** 19–26.

Cohen, J., and S. Honig (2005). "Anabolic steroid-associated infertility: A potentially treatable and reversible cause of male infertility." *Fertil and Steril* **84:** S223–S223.

Guzick, D. S., J. W. Overstreet, et al. (2001). "Sperm morphology, motility, and concentration in fertile and infertile men." *N Engl J Med* **345**(19): 1388–1393.

Hamed, S., K. Mohamed, et al. (2005). "The sexual and reproductive health in men with generalized epilepsy: A multidisciplinary evaluation." *Int J Impot Res* **18**(3): 287–295.

Keel, B. (2006). "Within- and between-subject variation in semen parameters in infertile men and normal semen donors." *Fertil and Steril* **85**(1): 128–134.

Keel, B. A. (2004). "How reliable are results from the semen analysis?" *Fertil and Steril* **82**(1): 41–44.

Lue, T. F. (2000). "Erectile dysfunction." *N Engl J Med* **342**(24): 1802–1813.

Ngo, A. D., R. Taylor, et al. (2006). "Association between Agent Orange and birth defects: Systematic review and meta-analysis." *Int J Epidemiol* **35**(5): 1220–1230.

Nieschlag, E. (2006). "Testosterone treatment comes of age: New options for hypogonadal men." *Clin Endocrinol* **65**(3): 275–281.

Perez, L. K., E. Titus, et al. (2005). "Reproductive outcomes in men with prenatal exposure to diethylstilbestrol." *Fertil and Steril* **84**(6): 1649–1656.

Sallmen, M., D. Sandler, et al. (2006). "Reduced fertility among overweight and obese men." *Epidemiol* **17**(5): 520–523.

Shores, M. M., A. M. Matsumoto, et al. (2006). "Low serum testosterone and mortality in male veterans." *Arch Intern Med* **166**(15): 1660–1665.

Simon, B., S. J. Lee, et al. (2005). "Preserving fertility after cancer." *CA Cancer J Clin* **55**(4): 211–228.

Steures, S. Van der, et al. (2005). "The value of the post-coital test in the basic fertility work-up: A nationwide cohort study and decision analysis." *Fertil and Steril* **84:** S358–S358.

Tielemans, E., R. van Kooij, et al. (2000). "Paternal occupational exposures and embryo implantation rates after IVF." *Fertil and Steril* **74**(4): 690–695.

Zhen, Q., X. Ye, et al. (1995). "Recent progress in research on tripterygium: A male antifertility plant." *Contraception* **51:** 117–120.

Chapter 9 ◆ Ovarian Factor

Al-Qahtani, A., and N. P. Groome (2006). "Anti-Müllerian hormone: Cinderella finds new admirers." *J Clin Endocrinol Metab* **91**(10): 3760–3762.

Amato, G., M. Conte, et al. (2003). "Serum and follicular fluid cytokines in polycystic ovary syndrome during stimulated cycles." *Obstet Gynecol* **101**(6): 1177–1182.

Andersen, C. Y., L. G. Westergaard, et al. (1993). "Endocrine composition of follicular fluid comparing human chorionic gonadotrophin to a gonadotrophin-releasing hormone agonist for ovulation induction." *Hum Reprod* **8**(6): 840–843.

Chavarro, J. E., J. W. Rich-Edwards, et al. (2006). "Iron intake and risk of ovulatory infertility." *Obstet Gynecol* **108**(5): 1145–1152.

Chavarro, J. E., J. W. Rich-Edwards, et al. (2007). "Dietary fatty acid intakes and the risk of ovulatory infertility." *Am J Clin Nutr* **85**(1): 231–237.

Dewailly, D., S. Catteau-Jonard, et al. (2006). "Oligoanovulation with polycystic ovaries but not overt hyperandrogenism." *J Clin Endocrinol Metab* **91**(10): 3922–3927.

Eldar-Geva, T., E. J. Margalioth, et al. (2002). "Serum inhibin B levels measured early during FSH administration for IVF may be of value in predicting the number of oocytes to be retrieved in normal and low responders." *Hum Reprod* **17**(9): 2331–2337.

Hendriks, D. J., F. J. M. Broekmans, et al. (2005). "Repeated clomiphene citrate challenge testing in the prediction of outcome in IVF: A comparison with basal markers for ovarian reserve." *Hum Reprod* **20**(1): 163–169.

Kezele, P. and M. K. Skinner (2003). "Regulation of ovarian primordial follicle assembly and development by estrogen and progesterone: Endocrine model of follicle assembly." *Endocrinol* **144**(8): 3329–3337.

La Marca, A., S. Giulini, et al. (2007). "Anti-Müllerian hormone measurement on any day of the menstrual cycle strongly predicts ovarian response in assisted reproductive technology." *Hum Reprod* **22**(3): 766–771.

Lannon, W. Von, et al. (2006). "Is follicular fluid steroid hormone content a marker of decreased fertility potential?" *Fertil and Steril* **86**(3): S388–S389.

Lobo, R. A. (2005). "Potential options for preservation of fertility in women." *N Engl J Med* **353**(1): 64–73.

McGovern, R. P., E. Legro, et al. (2007). "Utility of screening for other causes of infertility in women with "known" polycystic ovary syndrome." *Fertil and Steril* **87**(2): 442–444.

Murphy, M. K., J. E. Hall, et al. (2006). "Polycystic ovarian morphology in normal women does not predict the development of polycystic ovary syndrome." *J Clin Endocrinol Metab* **91**(10): 3878–3884.

Nilsson, E. E., C. Detzel, et al. (2006). "Platelet-derived growth factor modulates the primordial to primary follicle transition." *Reproduction* **131**(6): 1007–1015.

Pasquali, R., and A. Gambineri (2006). "Insulin-sensitizing agents in polycystic ovary syndrome." *Eur J Endocrinol* **154**(6): 763–775.

Simon, B., S. J. Lee, et al. (2005). "Preserving fertility after cancer." *CA Cancer J Clin* **55**(4): 211–228.

Srouji, S. S., Y. L. Pagan, et al. (2007). "Pharmacokinetic factors contribute to the inverse relationship between luteinizing hormone and body mass index in polycystic ovarian syndrome." *J Clin Endocrinol Metab* **92**(4): 1347–1352.

Visser, J. A., F. H. de Jong, et al. (2006). "Anti-Müllerian hormone: A new market for ovarian function." *Reproduction* **131**(1): 1–9.

Von Wald, T., B. Malizia, et al. (2006). "Specific peptide human follicular fluid composition correlates with age and fertility potential." *Obstet Gynecol* **107**(4) (Supplement): 9.

Welt, C. K., J. A. Gudmundsson, et al. (2006). "Characterizing discrete subsets of polycystic ovary syndrome as defined by the Rotterdam criteria: The impact of weight on phenotype and metabolic features." *J Clin Endocrinol Metab* **91**(12): 4842–4848.

Chapter 10 ◆ Tubal Factor

—. (2006). "Medical treatment of ectopic pregnancy." *Fertil and Steril* **86**(5): S96–S102.

—. (2006). "The role of tubal reconstructive surgery in the era of assisted reproductive technologies." *Fertil and Steril* **86**(5): S31–S34.

—. (2006). "Salpingectomy for hydrosalpinx prior to in vitro fertilization." *Fertil and Steril* **86**(5): S200–S201.

Al, F., Sylvestre, et al. (2006). "A randomized study of laparoscopic chromopertubation with lipiodol versus saline in infertile women." *Fertil and Steril* **85**(2): 505–507.

Awartani, K. and P. F. McComb (2003). "Microsurgical resection of nonocclusive salpingitis isthmica nodosa is beneficial." *Fertil and Steril* **79**(5): 1199–1203.

Baramki, T. (2005). "Hysterosalpingography." *Fertil and Steril* **83**(6): 1595–1606.

Gomel, V., and P. McComb (2006). "Microsurgery for tubal infertility." *J Reprod Med* **51**(3): 177–184.

Hubacher, D., D. Grimes, et al. (2004). "The limited clinical usefulness of taking a history in the evaluation of women with tubal factor infertility." *Fertil and Steril* **81**(1): 6–10.

Jamieson, D. J., S. C. Kaufman, et al. (2002). "A comparison of women's regret after vasectomy versus tubal sterilization." *Obstet Gynecol* **99**(6): 1073–1079.

Keltz, Gera, et al. (2006). "Chlamydia serology screening in infertility patients." *Fertil and Steril* **85**(3): 752–754.

Kontoravdis, E. A., K. Makrakis, et al. (2006). "Proximal tubal occlusion and salpingectomy result in similar improvement in in vitro fertilization outcome in patients with hydrosalpinx." *Fertil and Steril* **86**(6): 1642–1649.

Lin, P. C., K. P. Bhatnagar, et al. (2002). "Female genital anomalies affecting reproduction." *Fertil and Steril* **78**(5): 899–915.

O'Neill, C. (2005). "The role of paf in embryo physiology." *Hum Reprod Update* **11**(3): 215–228.

Ozmen, B., K. Diedrich, et al. (2007). "Hydrosalpinx and IVF: Assessment of treatments implemented prior to IVF." *Reprod BioMed Online* **14**: 235–241.

Renbaum, L., D. Ufberg, et al. (2002). "Reliability of clinicians versus radiologists for detecting abnormalities on hysterosalpingogram films." *Fertil and Steril* **78**(3): 614–618.

Roy, K., P. Hedge, et al. (2005). "Fimbrio-ovarian relationship in unexplained infertility." *Gynecol Obstet Invest* **60**(3): 128–132.

Chapter 11 ◆ Uterine Factor

—. (2006). "Myomas and reproductive function." *Fertil and Steril* **86**(5): S194–S199.

Giudice (2006). "Endometrium in PCOS: Implantation and predisposition to endocrine CA." *Best Pract & Res Clin Endocrinol & Metabol* **20**(2): 235–244.

Goldberg, J. M. and T. Falcone (1999). "Effect of diethylstilbestrol on reproductive function." *Fertil and Steril* **72**(1): 1–7.

Horcajadas, J. A., A. Pellicer, et al. (2007). "Wide genomic analysis of human endometrial receptivity: New times, new opportunities." *Hum Reprod Update* **13**(1): 77–86.

Khattab, S., I. Mohsen, et al. (2006). "Metformin reduces abortion in pregnant women with polycystic ovary syndrome." *Gynecol Endocrinol* **22**(12): 680–684.

E. Lamb (2004). "Looking at the endometrial biopsy with evidence-based medicine." *Fertil and Steril* **82**(5): 1283–1285.

Legro, R. R., L. Zaino, et al. (2007). "The effects of metformin and rosiglitazone, alone and in combination, on the ovary and endometrium in polycystic ovary syndrome." *Amer J Obstet and Gyn* **196**(4): 402.e1–402.e11.

Liberty, G., M. Gal, et al. (2007). "Lidocaine-prilocaine (EMLA) cream as analgesia for hysterosalpingography: A prospective, randomized, controlled, double blinded study." *Hum Reprod* **22**(5): 1335–1339.

Lin, P. C., K. P. Bhatnagar, et al. (2002). "Female genital anomalies affecting reproduction." *Fertil and Steril* **78**(5): 899–915.

Norwitz, E. R., D. J. Schust, et al. (2001). "Implantation and the survival of early pregnancy." *N Engl J Med* **345**(19): 1400–1408.

Oei, S. G., F. M. Helmerhorst, et al. (1998). "Effectiveness of the postcoital test: Randomised controlled trial." *BMJ* **317**(7157): 502–505.

Oppelt, H. von, et al. (2007). "Female genital malformations and their associated abnormalities." *Fertil and Steril* **87**(2): 335–342.

Soares, S. R., C. Simon, et al. (2007). "Cigarette smoking affects uterine receptiveness." *Hum Reprod* **22**(2): 543–547.

Strowitzki, T., A. Germeyer, et al. (2006). "The human endometrium as a fertility-determining factor." *Hum Reprod Update* **12**(5): 617–630.

Suarez, S. S. and A. A. Pacey (2006). "Sperm transport in the female reproductive tract." *Hum Reprod Update* **12**(1): 23–37.

Tur, K., Gal, et al. (2006). "A prospective evaluation of uterine abnormalities by saline infusion sonohysterography in 1,009 women with infertility or abnormal uterine bleeding." *Fertil and Steril* **86**(6): 1731–1735.

Chapter 12 ♦ Endometriosis and Recurrent Miscarriage

—. (2006). "Endometriosis and infertility." *Fertil and Steril* **86**(5): S156–S160.

—. (2006). "Intravenous immunoglobulin (IVIG) and recurrent spontaneous pregnancy loss." *Fertil and Steril* **86**(5): S226–S227.

Ballweg, M. L. (2005). "Selected food intake and risk of endometriosis." *Hum Reprod* **20**(1): 312–313.

Barnhart, K., R. Dunsmoor-Su, et al. (2002). "Effect of endometriosis on in vitro fertilization." *Fertil and Steril* **77**(6): 1148–1155.

Blount, B., J. Pirkle, et al. (2006). "Urinary perchlorate and thyroid hormone levels in adolescent and adult men and women living in the United States." *Environ Health Perspect* **114**(12): 1865–1871.

Buck Louis, G. M., J. M. Weiner, et al. (2005). "Environmental PCB exposure and risk of endometriosis." *Hum Reprod* **20**(1): 279–285.

Chapron, C., H. Barakat, et al. (2005). "Presurgical diagnosis of posterior deep infiltrating endometriosis based on a standardized questionnaire." *Hum Reprod* **20**(2): 507–513.

Christiansen, H. O., A. Nielsen, et al. (2006). "Inflammation and miscarriage." *Sem in Fetal and Neonat Med* **11**(5): 302–308.

Christiansen, H. O., A. Nybo, et al. (2005). "Evidence-based investigations and treatments of recurrent pregnancy loss." *Fertil and Steril* **83**(4): 821–839.

Cobellis, L., G. Latini, et al. (2003). "High plasma concentrations of di-(2-ethylhexyl)-phthalate in women with endometriosis." *Hum Reprod* **18**(7): 1512–1515.

D'Hooghe, T. M., and S. Debrock (2002). "Endometriosis, retrograde menstruation and peritoneal inflammation in women and in baboons." *Hum Reprod Update* **8**(1): 84–88.

Dewan, E. S., C. Puscheck, et al. (2006). "Y-chromosome microdeletions and recurrent pregnancy loss." *Fertil and Steril* **85**(2): 441–445.

Eskenazi, B., M. Warner, et al. (2001). "Validation study of nonsurgical diagnosis of endometriosis." *Fertil and Steril* **76**(5): 929–935.

Gao, O., et al. (2006). "Economic burden of endometriosis." *Fertil and Steril* **86**(6): 1561–1572.

Itsekson, A., D. Seidman, et al. (2007). "Recurrent pregnancy loss and inappropriate local immune response to sex hormones." *Am J Reprod Immun* **57**: 160–165.

Jackson, L. W., E. F. Schisterman, et al. (2005). "Oxidative stress and endometriosis." *Hum Reprod* **20**(7): 2014–2020.

Johns, J., E. Jauniaux, et al. (2006). "Factors affecting the early embryonic environment." *Rev Gynaecol and Perinat Prac* **6**: 199–210.

Khattab, S., I. A. Mohsen, et al. (2006). "Metformin reduces abortion in pregnant women with polycystic ovary syndrome." *Gynecol Endocrinol* **22**(12): 680–684.

Kogevinas, M. (2001). "Human health effects of dioxins: Cancer, reproductive and endocrine system effects." *Hum Reprod Update* **7**(3): 331–339.

Kohama, T., N. Suzuki, et al. (2004). "Analgesic efficacy of French maritime pine bark extract in dysmenorrhea: An open clinical trial." *J Reprod Med* **49**: 828–832.

Missmer, D. S., S. Spiegelman, et al. (2006). "Natural hair color and the incidence of endometriosis." *Fertil and Steril* **85**(4): 866–870.

Mojtaba Rezazadeh, V., K. Lila, et al. (2006). "Efficacy of a human embryo transfer medium: A prospective, randomized clinical trial study." *J Assist Reprod and Genet* **23**(5): 207–212.

Nardo, L., and H. Saliam (2006). "Progesterone supplementation to prevent recurrent miscarriage and to reduce implantation failure in assisted reproduction cycles." *Reprod BioMed Online* **13**(1): 47–57.

Parazzini, F., F. Chiaffarino, et al. (2004). "Selected food intake and risk of endometriosis." *Hum Reprod* **19**(8): 1755–1759.

Pauwels, A., P. J. C. Schepens, et al. (2001). "The risk of endometriosis and exposure to dioxins and polychlorinated biphenyls: A case-control study of infertile women." *Hum Reprod* **16**(10): 2050–2055.

Poppe, K., B. Velkeniers, et al. (2007). "Thyroid disease and female reproduction." *Clin Endocrinol* **66**(3): 309–321.

Porter, T., and J. Scott (2005). "Evidence-based care of recurrent miscarriage." *Best Prac & Res Clin Obstet & Gynaecol* **19**(1): 85–101.

Quenby, K., et al. (2005). "Prednisolone reduces preconceptual endometrial natural killer cells in women with recurrent miscarriage." *Fertil and Steril* **84**(4): 980–984.

Raber, W., P. Nowotny, et al. (2003). "Thyroxine treatment modified in infertile women according to thyroxine-releasing hormone testing: 5 year follow-up of 283 women referred after exclusion of absolute causes of infertility." *Hum Reprod* **18**(4): 707–714.

Rai, R., and L. Regan (2006). "Recurrent miscarriage." *Lancet* **368**(9535): 601–611.

Rier, S., and W. G. Foster (2002). "Environmental dioxins and endometriosis." *Toxicol Sci* **70**(2): 161–170.

Rier, S. E. (2002). "The potential role of exposure to environmental toxicants in the pathophysiology of endometriosis." *Ann NY Acad Sci* **955**(1): 201–212.

Sharpe, R. M., and D. S. Irvine (2004). "How strong is the evidence of a link between environmental chemicals and adverse effects on human reproductive health?" *BMJ* **328**(7437): 447–451.

Soares, S., C. Simon, et al. (2007). "Cigarette smoking affects uterine receptiveness." *Hum Reprod* **22**(2): 543–547.

Stephenson, M. D., and M. H. H. Ensom (2002). "An update on the role of immunotherapy in reproductive failure." *Immunol and Allerg Clin of North Amer* **22**(3): 623–642.

Stricker, R. B., A. Steinleitner, et al. (2002). "Intravenous immunoglobulin (IVIG) therapy for immunologic abortion." *Clin and App Immunol Rev* **2**(3): 187–199.

Sugiura-Ogasawara, M., Y. Ozaki, et al. (2005). "Exposure to bisphenol A is associated with recurrent miscarriage." *Hum Reprod* **20**(8): 2325–2329.

Welshons, W. V., S. C. Nagel, et al. (2006). "Large effects from small exposures. III. endocrine mechanisms mediating effects of bisphenol A at levels of human exposure." *Endocrinol* **147**(6): S56–69.

Chapter 13 ◆ Basic Reproductive Treatment

—. (2004). "Guidelines for the provision of infertility services." *Fertil and Steril* **82:** 24–25.

—. (2006). "Multiple pregnancy associated with infertility therapy." *Fertil and Steril* **86**(5): S106–S110.

—. (2006). "Ovarian hyperstimulation syndrome." *Fertil and Steril* **86**(5): S178–S183.

—. (2006). "2006 Guidelines for gamete and embryo donation." *Fertil and Steril* **86**(5): S38–S50.

—. (2006). "Use of clomiphene citrate in women." *Fertil and Steril* **86**(5): S187–S193.

Bachelot, A., and N. Binart (2007). "Reproductive role of prolactin." *Reproduction* **133**(2): 361–369.

Branigan, E. F., and M. A. Estes (2003). "A randomized clinical trial of treatment of clomiphene citrate–resistant anovulation with the use of oral contraceptive pill suppression and repeat clomiphene citrate treatment." *Amer J Obstet and Gynecol* **188**(6): 1424–1430.

Carroll, N., and J. R. Palmer (2001). "A comparison of intrauterine versus intracervical insemination in fertile single women." *Fertil and Steril* **75**(4): 656–660.

Casadei, Z., et al. (2006). "Homologous intrauterine insemination in controlled ovarian hyperstimulation cycles: A comparison among three different regimens." *Europ J Obstet and Gynecol* **129**(2): 155–161.

Dumesic, D. A., T. G. Lesnick, et al. (2007). "Increased adiposity enhances intrafollicular estradiol levels in normoandrogenic ovulatory women receiving gonadotropin-releasing hormone analog/recombinant human follicle-stimulating hormone therapy for in vitro fertilization." *J Clin Endocrinol Metab* **92**(4): 1438–1441.

Freeman, G., et al. (2007). "Association of anti-Müllerian hormone levels with obesity in late reproductive-age women." *Fertil and Steril* **87**(1): 101–106.

Guzick, D. S. (2007). "Treating the polycystic ovary syndrome the old-fashioned way." *N Engl J Med* **356**(6): 622–624.

Haebe, J., J. Martin, et al. (2002). "Success of intrauterine insemination in women aged 40–42 years." *Fertil and Steril* **78**(1): 29–33.

Holzer, R. H., T. Casper, et al. (2006). "A new era in ovulation induction." *Fertil and Steril* **85**(2): 277–284.

Ibericolbérico, G., J. Vioque, et al. (2004). "Analysis of factors influencing pregnancy rates in homologous intrauterine insemination." *Fertil and Steril* **81**(5): 1308–1313.

Jones (2007). "Iatrogenic multiple births: A 2003 checkup." *Fertil and Steril* **87**(3): 453–455.

Legro, R. S., H. X. Barnhart, et al. (2007). "Clomiphene, metformin, or both for infertility in the polycystic ovary syndrome." *N Engl J Med* **356**(6): 551–566.

Mitwally, M. F., B. Biljan, et al. (2005). "Pregnancy outcome after the use of an aromatase inhibitor for ovarian stimulation." *Amer J Obstet and Gynecol* **192**(2): 381–386.

Osuna, C., R. Matorras, et al. (2004). "One versus two inseminations per cycle in intrauterine insemination with sperm from patients' husbands: A systematic review of the literature." *Fertil and Steril* **82**(1): 17–24.

Poppe, K., B. Velkeniers, et al. (2007). "Thyroid disease and female reproduction." *Clin Endocrinol* **66**(3): 309–321.

Ryan, G. L., S. H. Zhang, et al. (2004). "The desire of infertile patients for multiple births." *Fertil and Steril* **81**(3): 500–504.

Stener-Victorin, E., M. Wikland, et al. (2002). "Alternative treatments in reproductive medicine: Much ado about nothing: Acupuncture—a method of treatment in reproductive medicine: Lack of evidence of an effect does not equal evidence of the lack of an effect." *Hum Reprod* **17**(8): 1942–1946.

Chapter 14 ◆ Advanced Reproductive Treatments

—. (2006). "Ovarian hyperstimulation syndrome." *Fertil and Steril* **86**(5): S178–S183.

—. (2006). "2006 Guidelines for gamete and embryo donation." *Fertil and Steril* **86**(5): S38–S50.

—. (2007). "ACOG Committee Opinion No. 360: Sex selection." *Obstet Gynecol* **109**(2): 475–478.

Abusief, M., T. Hornstein, et al. (2007). "Assessment of United States fertility clinic websites according to the American Society for Reproductive Medicine (ASRM)/Society for Assisted Reproductive Technology (SART) guidelines." *Fertil and Steril* **87**(1): 88–92.

Bellver, J., C. Busso, et al. (2006). "Obesity and assisted reproductive technology outcomes." *Reprod BioMed Online* **12**: 562–568.

Buckett, W. M. (2003). "A meta-analysis of ultrasound-guided versus clinical touch embryo transfer." *Fertil and Steril* **80**(4): 1037–1041.

Collins, J. A. (2002). "An international survey of the health economics of IVF and ICSI." *Hum Reprod Update* **8**(3): 265–277.

Geber, S., A. C. F. Moreira, et al. (2007). "Comparison between two forms of vaginally administered progesterone for luteal phase support in assisted reproduction cycles." *Reprod BioMed Online* **14**: 155–158.

Ives, A., C. Saunders, et al. (2007). "Pregnancy after breast cancer: Population based study." *BMJ* **334**(7586): 194.

Lambers, M. J., E. Mager, et al. (2007). "Factors determining early pregnancy loss in singleton and multiple implantations." *Hum Reprod* **22**(1): 275–279.

Makrakis, E., J. Angeli, et al. (2006). "Laser versus mechanical assisted hatching: A prospective study of clinical outcomes." *Fertil and Steril* **86**(6): 1596–1600.

Olson, N., Keppler, et al. (2005). "In vitro fertilization is associated with an increase in major birth defects." *Fertil and Steril* **84**(5): 1308–1315.

Papanikolaou, E. G., M. Camus, et al. (2006). "In vitro fertilization with single blastocyst-stage versus single cleavage-stage embryos." *N Engl J Med* **354**(11): 1139–1146.

Reddy, U. M., R. J. Wapner, et al. (2007). "Infertility, assisted reproductive technology, and adverse pregnancy outcomes: Executive summary of a national institute of child health and human development workshop." *Obstet Gynecol* **109**(4): 967–977.

Richter, K., K. Bugge, et al. (2007). "Relationship between endometrial thickness and embryo implantation, based on 1,294 cycles of in vitro fertilization with transfer of two blastocyst-stage embryos." *Fertil and Steril* **87**(1): 53–59.

Schieve, L. A. (2006). "The promise of single-embryo transfer." *N Engl J Med* **354**(11): 1190–1193.

Schwarzler, P., H. Zech, et al. (2004). "Pregnancy outcome after blastocyst transfer as compared to early cleavage stage embryo transfer." *Hum Reprod* **19**(9): 2097–2102.

Shamonki, M. I., S. D. Spandorfer, et al. (2005). "Ultrasound-guided embryo transfer and the accuracy of trial embryo transfer." *Hum Reprod* **20**(3): 709–716.

Silber, S. J., and R. G. Gosden (2007). "Ovarian transplantation in a series of monozygotic twins discordant for ovarian failure." *N Engl J Med* **356**(13): 1382–1384.

Spandorfer, S., K. Bendikson, et al. (2007). "Outcome of in vitro fertilization in women 45 years and older who use autologous oocytes." *Fertil and Steril* **87**(1): 74–76.

Thurin, A., J. Hausken, et al. (2004). "Elective single-embryo transfer versus double-embryo transfer in in vitro fertilization." *N Engl J Med* **351**(23): 2392–2402.

Tian, L., H. Shen, et al. (2007). "Insulin resistance increases the risk of spontaneous abortion following assisted reproduction technology treatment." *J Clin Endocrinol Metab:* **92**(4): 1430–1433.

Toner, J. P. (2002). "Progress we can be proud of: U.S. trends in assisted reproduction over the first 20 years." *Fertil and Steril* **78**(5): 943–950.

van der Gaast, M. H., M. J. C. Eijkemans, et al. (2006). "Optimum number of oocytes for a successful first IVF treatment cycle." *Reprod BioMed Online* **13**: 476–480.

Van Voorhis, B. J. (2007). "In vitro fertilization." *N Engl J Med* **356**(4): 379–386.

Verhaak, C. M., J. M. J. Smeenk, et al. (2007). "Women's emotional adjustment to IVF: A systematic review of 25 years of research." *Hum Reprod Update* **13**(1): 27–36.

Conclusion ◆ Taking Action

Bates, B. (2004). "Fear of failure deters many from infertility Tx." *Ob Gyn News* **39**(15): 20.

Greene, R., and L. Tarkan (2007). *Dr. Robert Greene's Perfect Hormone Balance for Pregnancy.* New York, Three Rivers Press.

Reynolds, M. A., L. A. Schieve, et al. (2003). "Does insurance coverage decrease the risk for multiple births associated with assisted reproductive technology?" *Fertil and Steril* **80**(1): 16–23.

ACKNOWLEDGMENTS

I've scoured the latest research to put together this information into a practical program that you would find useful and easy to follow. But I didn't do it alone. So let me introduce and acknowledge the incredible team that was involved in creating this book, which I hope will change your life forever.

I first want to express my deepest gratitude to my wife, Morgan Pritchard. When she agreed to include our personal experience as a couple seeking pregnancy, I was surprised and delighted. She is a very private person, but she chose to share such an intimate aspect of our life to help encourage and inspire others as they try to become pregnant. In addition to our profile, her fingerprints can be found throughout this book, especially in the great lists, charts, and tables. She truly is my partner in all things, including this book.

My writing partner, Laurie Tarkan, continues to be insightful, inspiring, and invaluable. She has done wonders to organize, translate, and explain the latest science. I remain in awe of her. Her perspective and voice blend well with my own. As a result of our collaboration, you're getting a much broader perspective beyond what I could have offered alone. I'd also like to thank her husband, Andrew Lipetz, for tolerating the disruption that three books written in succession has had upon their home life.

My agent, Stedman Mays of Scribblers House, continues to guide me through the publishing world. His meticulous attention to detail and riotous laugh are only a few of his endearing assets. More than just an agent, he is truly a friend and ally. Thanks, Sted.

I must also express my appreciation to Amy Pierpont, our discerning and sagacious editor. I look forward to working with you on future projects. I'd also like to thank her abettor, Lindsay Miller. You kept me out of trouble on more than one occasion and were always quick to answer my nagging questions.

The Crown Publishing Group is the best. They've shared the vision of Perfect Hormone Balance and patiently facilitated this work. To Lauren Shakely, Jenny Frost, and Pam Krauss, I want to express a very special "thank-you" for giving me this chance to empower so many to become parents.

Tina Constable, Annsley Rosner, and Melanie DeNardo are the greatest promotional team any author could hope for. Their persistence and support means the world to me. Thanks for getting this information out there and recognized.

Our production editor, Cindy Berman, kept this book moving smoothly from manuscript through the steps of composition and copyediting. Doris Cooper and Carrie Thornton are the wonderful editorial directors who oversaw publication. The artistic team that put a face on this book, including the cover design, was Dominika Dmytrowski, Jane Treuhaft, and Marysarah Quinn. Great job.

Sometimes words alone aren't enough. Luckily, we had the assistance of Gail Tarkan Shube, who saved us several thousand words with her illustrations. I'm very grateful for your contribution.

Finally, I want to thank all of the many wonderful patients that have taught me so much over the last 15 years. It's because of you that I created this program. Most of the information in this book isn't taught at any medical school. It was learned through listening to and melding your experience with the emerging research. You've helped so many and continue to enhance my knowledge and perspective as well. Thank you all.

—ROBERT

◆　◆　◆

I would like to express my gratitude to the Tarkan, Lipetz, and Shube families, who have been so supportive of my writing. A giant hug goes to my children, Miranda and Jordan, for trying to understand why I worked such long hours for so long. And to my husband, Andrew Lipetz, thank you for all your support, faith, and love. I also want to thank my amazing friends, who were incredibly patient as I disappeared for months on end to complete this book and who were supportive and encouraging when I needed them—thank you Karen Nielsen, Hilary Macht, Linda Caporaletti, and Lisa Basile. Always a special thanks to Lynne Cusack, my good friend and mentor.

I wish to thank my agent, Stedman Mays of Scribblers House, for pairing me up with Robert and for this great writing experience. Your encouragement and calming words of wisdom continue to keep me on an even keel through the harder moments of writing. I'm grateful to our editor, Amy Pierpont, whose inquisitive mind, keen eye for detail, and smart editing has helped bring depth and clarity to this book. I'd like to thank Morgan Pritchard, who provided me with editorial and especially moral support, and who has become a great friend. Many thanks to the team at the Crown Publishing Group for all your efforts to usher this book through production. And a special thank-you to my sister, Gail Tarkan Shube, for drawing the wonderful illustrations in this book.

And thank you, Robert, for allowing me to continue to be your writing partner. I greatly admire your mission to educate couples struggling with fertility, and am honored to be a part of it.

—LAURIE

INDEX

ABOUT THE AUTHORS

Robert A. Greene received his medical degree from Ohio State University. He completed his internship and residency in obstetrics and gynecology at the University of Louisville and continued on to a subspecialty fellowship in reproductive endocrinology and infertility at Harbor-UCLA Medical Center. Dr. Greene is board-certified in both his specialty and subspecialty. He serves as the medical director of the Sher Institute for Reproductive Medicine in Northern California, where he offers comprehensive evaluation and individualized fertility treatment. He also treats a wide variety of generalized hormonal disorders in both men and women. His practice style combines equal parts compassion, cutting-edge science, and patient empowerment.

Dr Greene's research involving various aspects of the hormone brain connection has been published in prestigious medical journals, including *Fertility & Sterility, The Female Patient, OB/GYN Clinics of North America,* and *The Aging Male.* He has become a go-to expert on hormone balance and frequently lectures to health-care providers throughout the United States and internationally in Europe, Japan, Singapore, and South America. Based on his years of experience, he developed a fully integrative approach to diagnosing and treating problems related to hormone imbalance, especially as they relate to pregnancy and infertility. He has authored several books dedicated to providing comprehensive, evidence-based information about diet, lifestyle, environmental toxins, supplements, and complementary medicine, as well as the latest in BioIdentical hormone intervention.

Dr. Greene lives and works in Northern California with his wife and daughter. If you or your health-care provider would like additional information to correct your hormone balance or treat your fertility problem, check out his website at www.RobertGreeneMD.com.

◆　◆　◆

Laurie Tarkan is an award-winning medical journalist who writes frequently for the *New York Times*. She is the author of *My Mother's Breast: Daughters Face Their Mothers' Cancer* (Taylor Trade Publishing, 1999) and the coauthor of *Dr. Robert Greene's Perfect Hormone Balance for Pregnancy* and *Happy Baby, Healthy Mom Pregnancy Journal*. She has written about health and women's issues for national consumer magazines, including *Glamour, Health, Parenting, Self, Child, Fit Pregnancy,* and *Family Circle.*

ALSO BY ROBERT A. GREENE, M.D.

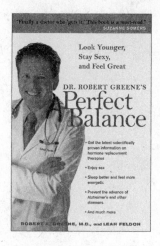

Dr. Robert Greene's
Perfect Balance

Look Younger, Stay Sexy, and Feel Great

$14.95 paper (Canada: $21.00)
978-0-307-33620-0

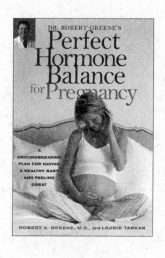

Dr. Robert Greene's
Perfect Hormone Balance
for Pregnancy

A Groundbreaking Plan for Having
a Healthy Baby and Feeling Great

$15.95 paper (Canada: $19.95)
978-0-307-33738-2

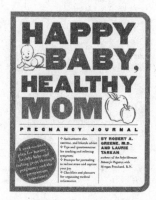

Happy Baby, Healthy Mom
Pregnancy Journal

Robert A. Greene, M.D., and Laurie Tarkan

A Week-to-Week Plan for Having
a Healthy Baby and Feeling Great through
Pregnancy and the Postpartum Experience

$18.95 paper-over-board (Canada: $24.95)
978-0-307-38221-4

Available wherever books are sold.